Hemoglobin-based Red Cell Substitutes

The Johns Hopkins Series in Contemporary Medicine and Public Health

Also of interest in this series

J. David Bessman, M.D., *Automated Blood Counts and Differentials: A Practical Guide*

Horst Brücher, M.D., *Bone Marrow Diagnosis in Clinical Practice*

Emmanuel N. Dessypris, M.D., *Pure Red Cell Aplasia*

Allan J. Erslev, M.D., D.Sc., John W. Adamson, M.D., Joseph W. Eschbach, M.D., and Christopher G. Winearls, M.B., Ch.B., D.Phil., eds., *Erythropoietin: Molecular, Cellular, and Clinical Biology*

R. Madhok, M.D., C. D. Forbes, M.D., and B. L. Evatt, M.D., eds., *Blood, Blood Products, and AIDS*

George Stamatoyannopoulos, M.D., and Arthur W. Nienhuis, M.D., eds., *The Regulation of Hemoglobin Switching*

Robert M. Winslow, M.D., and Carlos Monge C., M.D., *Hypoxia, Polycythemia, and Chronic Mountain Sickness*

Hemoglobin-based Red Cell Substitutes

Robert M. Winslow, M.D.
Chief, Blood Research Division
Letterman Army Institute of Research, San Francisco
and
Adjunct Professor, Department of Medicine
University of California, San Diego

The Johns Hopkins University Press
Baltimore and London

Printed in the United States of America

The Johns Hopkins University Press, 701 West 40th Street
Baltimore, Maryland 21211-2190
The Johns Hopkins Press Ltd., London

∞ The paper used in this book meets the minimum requirements of American National Standard for Information Sciences—Permanence of Paper for Printed Library Materials, ANSI Z39.48-1984.

Library of Congress Cataloging-in-Publication Data

Winslow, Robert M., 1941–
Hemoglobin-based red cell substitutes / Robert M. Winslow.
p. cm.—(The Johns Hopkins series in contemporary medicine and public health)
Includes bibliographical references and index.
ISBN 0-8018-4245-X (alk. paper)
1. Blood substitutes. 2. Hemoglobin. I. Title. II. Series.
[DNLM: 1. Blood Substitutes. WH 450 W781h]
RM171.7.W56 1992
615′.39—dc20
DNLM/DLC
for Library of Congress 91-7098

Contents

Preface

On March 14, 1990, an unusual meeting was held on the campus of the National Institutes of Health which will surely set the course for development of red cell substitutes over the next few years, if not longer. The meeting, jointly sponsored by the Food and Drug Administration, the National Institutes of Health, and the U.S. Army Medical Research and Development Command, aimed to sift through the existing data on clinical trials of hemoglobin-based red cells substitutes in an effort to establish guidelines for further human studies. Representatives from each of the commercial manufacturers of hemoglobin derivatives were asked to present their views and data on the safety of their products. In addition, some of the information offered in this book was presented as a review of past progress and a statement of the current status of the field.

After discussion of the published and unpublished data concerning the solutions under development, the Blood Products Advisory Committee (with several consultants) issued a public statement outlining suggested studies to establish safety standards for candidate solutions. This statement was perceived by some to be excessively stringent, requiring experiments that were overly detailed and expensive. As reflected in the popular press (*Business Week,* May 21, 1990, pp. 42–43), some members of the business community felt these recommendations represented a serious setback to the field. However, the meeting underscored the complexity of the problem of developing a safe red cell substitute, and in fact the recommendations of this panel formed a blueprint for continued development.

The complex interplay of scientific discipline, industry, and clinical medicine can be bewildering. However, successful integration will present new opportunities, and involvement of young scientists is essential to progress in the field. My principal motivation in writing this book was to present the state of the field, in historical perspective, in a concise way so that those new to the field can have a ready source of information.

In preparation of this manuscript, I reviewed more than 1200 articles in the literature. Less than half are cited, and I take complete responsibility for the selection. I have tried to cite only those sources that present key data or express innovative points of view. Because this is a multidisciplinary field, most readers will find some chapters more tedious or more interesting than others. It was especially difficult to arrange the sequence of the chapters. For example, Chapter 2 introduces clinical applications before the details of the biochemical and physiologic properties are discussed. Some readers may wish to read the chapters in a different sequence, depending on their interests. The last chapter, although somewhat redundant, contains a short summary of all of the preceding chapters. Some readers might wish to read this chapter first for an overall flavor of the book.

The content of the book necessarily reflects my own biases even though I have attempted to avoid the appearance of favoring one approach or product over another. Furthermore, I have used examples from our own work at the Letterman Army Institute of Research liberally because it is convenient to do so; data from other laboratories could have been used to make many of the same points. This is a field in rapid change, and it is certain that there will be oversights and omissions. It would be impossible to summarize progress without offending some who have made important contributions. To them I apologize; the views presented here are my own and do not necessarily reflect the official opinions of the U.S. Army or the Department of Defense.

I would like to thank my colleagues in the Blood Research Division, Letterman Army Institute of Research, for their stimulation and patience. Drs. Everse, Hess, Keipert, Kim, Macdonald, Marks, Marini, McFaul, Moore, Panter, and Vandegriff have shared the adventure for the past several years. Val Coppes, Mike Cross, Yvonne LeTellier, Ron Fishman, Edith Moore, Alison Murray, Dan Smith, Ed Wood, and Angelo Zegna have contributed expert technical assistance to all of us, as have the many fine young enlisted soldiers who have served in the division: Rob Jesse, Shawn Snell, Jerry Knopp, and Keith Lamay. Vonceal Johnson has spent many long hours in the enormous task of collecting bibliographic material. I owe a special debt of gratitude to Keith Chapman, whose contribution to all phases of our work was indispensable; to Mike French, who helped organize our production facility; and, as always, to my family, for their amazing tolerance. I would like to acknowledge the special place in our lives of our late colleagues and friends, Mr. Frank Medina and Col. Ed Beatrice. But most of all, this book is for Sally.

Introduction

Red cell substitutes are solutions intended for use in patients who need red cell transfusions, for which either red cells are not available or their use is to be avoided for other reasons. More than one hundred years of research have not produced a solution that can be used safely in humans. Amberson, reviewing the progress on red cell substitutes up until 1937, observed that although the practice of infusing milk in the absence of blood had been abandoned, Ringer-Locke solution, which contains hemoglobin, was a very promising resuscitation solution and that "a substitute for blood has become one of the most pressing needs of the experimental laboratory" (Amberson 1937). More than fifty years later many of the problems Amberson outlined have been solved, but many others remain.

Why have red cell substitutes not fulfilled the promise envisioned by early workers? One obvious reason is that their development is an extremely ambitious goal. Another is that few have shared Amberson's view of their need: at the same time that Amberson was working on the problem, blood banking technology was developing at a rapid pace, and it appeared that there was really no need, on a large scale, for a red cell substitute. Much of the motivation for the early work in the field must have come from the simple desire to understand the relative importance of the various components of human blood. Thus, red cell substitutes have not attracted the attention of a large number of scientists.

World War II led to the maturation of the blood banking system, and human albumin was prepared and packaged for the military for use on the battlefield. In the Korean and Vietnamese conflicts, human blood was available in reasonable supply, and although it seems intuitively obvious that an oxygen-carrying colloid solution would be superior to one that does not carry oxygen, no direct evidence was available and no products seemed to be on the horizon. The military has continued to support research and development of blood substitutes of all types, but the number of investigators working in the field has been small and progress painfully slow.

In 1983 attention to development of red cell substitutes intensified when it was recognized that the acquired immune deficiency syndrome (AIDS) could be transmitted by a blood-borne virus (HIV). National hysteria concerning the nation's blood supply followed. Anemic patients refused to receive blood transfusions, and health care workers panicked at the possibility of contracting the disease from casual contact with AIDS patients or blood collected from them. Many surgeons and operating room personnel became alarmed at the prospect of contact with banked blood.

In this context, research into red cell substitutes entered a new phase and became clearly dependent on the availability of carefully prepared study material. The AIDS epidemic drew industry into the field because of the enormous implied market. Financial support for red cell substitute research was increasingly available from the National Heart, Lung, and Blood Institute and from the U.S. Army, the Navy, and from private sources.

As new capital poured into efforts to commercialize red cell substitute products, many scientists entered the field for the first time. Veterans of classic areas of medical research found new life in investigations into the biochemistry, biology, and physiology of red cell substitutes. Molecular biology, too, has made contributions to the field as hemoglobin can now be expressed in bacteria, yeast, and transgenic animals, and site-directed mutants provide important new insight into hemoglobin function. Younger investigators now feel that red cell substitutes is a field of its own. Gradually, in the past five years, new light has been shed on some of the problems in this field; but the enthusiasm of a decade ago has faded somewhat as new problems are encountered.

AIDS has had a positive impact on transfusion practice. Other retroviruses have been identified, efforts to screen blood not only for these agents but also for viruses that cause hepatitis have intensified, the indications for transfusion have been reevaluated, and the use of blood products has become much more efficient. More careful screening of donors, testing of all donated units, and a general awareness in the donor population have all contributed to a decreased risk from transfusion AIDS since 1983.

These developments should lead to more prudent, realistic development of products. As the nation's blood supply becomes safer and indications for transfusion more conservative, the perceived profitability of potential products may diminish. Eventually, I believe, oxygen-carrying solutions, based on hemoglobin in some form, will take their place in the therapeutic armamentarium. To predict what their uses will be or in what volume they would be used is premature at this time.

Chapter 1
Historical Background

In his 1937 review on blood substitutes, Amberson wrote,

> The blood of vertebrates is the most complicated fluid to be found in the world of living organisms. Compounded of a dozen essential ingredients, sustaining a multiplicity of activities, the fluid pathway for a variety of chemical and hormonal integrations of function, the source of food and oxygen for every tissue, it defies laboratory synthesis. At the very beginning we must recognize that there is no complete substitute for blood. Yet biologists and physiologists, no less than clinicians, are so frequently confronted with situations where normal blood cannot be obtained, or where the problem at issue can only be solved by a simplification of conditions, that a substitute for blood has become one of the most pressing needs of the experimental laboratory.

More than fifty years later there is still no substitute for blood to be used for transfusion in spite of substantial efforts to produce one. This chapter will review some developments in transfusion medicine which relate to red cell substitutes and will present some of the forces that have driven research in the field. At the outset, the obvious may be stated: if it were a simple problem, it would have been solved long ago.

The U. S. Army, which contributed so much to the blood-banking system and to the development of human serum albumin as a therapeutic agent, has long recognized the impact that a universal oxygen-carrying resuscitation fluid would have in the care of trauma victims. Wartime requirements placed the military in the center of research and development efforts, and now the military is a certain market for red cell substitute products. Work on such solutions has been carried out in both military and civilian laboratories for the more than twenty years since it was discovered that hemoglobin could be modified chemically to improve its usefulness as a cell-free oxygen carrier.

Efforts to develop products for nonmilitary use have intensified recently for several reasons. First, the supply of blood for transfusion in the United States is diminishing. This arises from a combination of more efficient usage of banked blood and the fear of many potential donors that the act of donation might expose them to viral infection. Second, the acquired immune-deficiency syndrome (AIDS) epidemic has made both physicians and patients aware that there is an inherent risk in receiving banked blood. Third, efforts to control the human immunodeficiency virus (HIV) have drawn attention to other pathogenic viruses that can potentially contaminate blood. Finally, scientists are becoming increasingly aware of the possibility of turning their efforts to profit.

Frequently when a research area does not fulfill its promise, the reasons lie in the fact that related fields are also relatively undeveloped, and fundamental insights into basic biologic mechanisms are lacking (Comroe 1976). Such is the nature of the red cell substitute problem. Ever since William Harvey described blood circulation in 1628 a red cell substitute has seemed nearly at hand. Nevertheless by 1990 only four clinical trials with hemoglobin-based red cell substitutes had been carried out. Two of them have not been published. One, a tolerance study, was so limited that few clinical conclusions may be drawn from it. Two were conducted outside of the United States, and the data have never been published.

1.1 A Brief History of Blood Transfusion

The histories of blood transfusion and red cell substitutes are complementary: without a need for transfusions, there would be no need for alternatives. More than three hundred years passed between the first description of blood circulation in the body and the implementation of routine transfusion in medicine. It is not surprising that a little more time is needed to develop safe, practical red cell substitutes (Table 1.1).

1.1.1 Early Studies

The lore of blood transfusion is rooted in antiquity. Leviticus 7:26, which forbids the eating of blood, is the basis today for the refusal by certain religious groups to receive transfusions. But the ancient Egyptians used "blood baths" as a restorative, and Romans apparently rushed into the arenas to drink the blood of dying gladiators. However, no transfusion could occur until the circulation of the blood was understood.

Although Ibn Nafis described the pulmonary circulation in the thirteenth century (Comroe 1976), William Harvey described his theory of the circulation of the blood independently in 1616 and published his views in 1628 for the first time in the Western literature (Harvey 1653). Harvey had been trained in Padua to acquire knowledge by direct observation, a method he used to great advantage in England (Dormandy 1978). His magnificent contribution to science was the key that opened the door to modern studies of blood transfusion, and almost immediately after its publication, efforts in the quest for red cell substitutes began.

Table 1.1. The History of Blood Substitutes

Year	Event
1628	Circulation of the blood (Harvey)
1656	Wine, scammony, opium, blood (Wren)
1665	First animal transfusion (Lower)
1667	First human transfusion (Denis), death, moratorium
1818	Renewed interest in transfusion (Blundell)
1835	Defibrination of blood (Bischoff)
1863	Gum-saline (Ludwig)
1867	Bacteria, fungi, asepsis (Pasteur; LIster)
1871	Plasma and serum
1878	MIlk, cholera epidemic (Thomas; Jennings; Hodder; Bovell)
1900	Red cell antigens (Landsteiner)
1916	Hemoglobin infusions in humans (Sellards and Minot)
1937	Amberson's review
1941–45	Albumin, hemoglobin
1949	Amberson's report of hemoglobin infusions in humans
1957	Encapsulated hemoglobin (Chang)
1966	"Bloodless" mouse (Clark and Gollan)
1967	PFC emulsion (Sloviter and Kamimoto)
1967	Stroma-free hemoglobin (Rabiner et al.)
1968	Exchange transfusion with PFC (Geyer, Monroe, and Taylor)
1968	Hemoglobin dimerization demonstrated (Bunn and Jandl)
1972	Modification to reduce oxygen affinity (Benesch et al.)
1973	Glutaraldehyde polymerization (Payne)
1976	"Polyhemoglobin" (Bonhard)
1978	Human safety trial, unmodified hemoglobin (Savitsky et al.)
1989	Human trials with "polyhemoglobin" (Moss et al.)

The first successful blood transfusion from one animal to another was probably performed in 1665 by Richard Lower and Edmund King (Hollingsworth 1928). Such early efforts used the quills of bird feathers to puncture arteries or veins, and blood was collected in animal bladders. Not surprisingly, there were many failures! It is of interest that Lower's experiments were directed at perfecting the technique of injection with various solutions such as wines and beers. In the course of his experiments he noted that these solutions mixed freely with blood but not when mixed ex vivo. Therefore, to test their miscibility, he injected them intravenously (Hollingsworth 1928).

Lower's success captured the imagination of the Royal Society of London, and he received widespread attention for it. There was rampant speculation on the question of whether a dog would grow wool, hoofs and horns after transfusion with sheep's blood. Samuel Pepys speculated that the new practice of transfusion "did give rise to many pretty wishes, as of the blood of a Quaker to be let into an Archbishop and such like" (Nicolson 1965). It was also proposed that the phlegmatic personality could be corrected by transfusion with blood from a choleric and even that marital discord could be settled by reciprocal transfusion of husband and wife.

One important observation was also made by Pepys: "Above all I was pleased to see the person who had his blood taken out. He speaks well, and did this day give the Society a relation thereof in Latin, saying that he finds himself much better since, and as a new man." Apparently there was some concern that the act of blood donation was not safe.

Although one romantic story describes the collection of blood from three boys to transfuse into Pope Innocent VIII in 1492 (Lindboom 1954), the first human transfusions were actually performed in France. Perhaps the first successful one was the work of Jean Baptiste Denis, the physician to Louis XIV, in June 1667. A young boy who suffered from an obscure illness and had been treated by venesection to the point of exhaustion received a small amount of lamb's blood and made a remarkable recovery. In the wake of this success, Denis transfused additional patients until one, upon receipt of a third transfusion, died, apparently because of an incompatibility reaction. Denis was charged with murder but was eventually exonerated. This experience, and the publicity it stirred, led to a moratorium on transfusion practice in France, England, and Italy, and research abated.

The search for a red cell substitute paralleled the search for safe blood transfusion. In retrospect, both quests were doomed because of the need for basic advances in related fields. Initially, however, it was thought that transfusion of blood was completely unsafe and that only alternatives could be used. Therefore the eventual need for a substitute decreased when safe transfusion practices became available.

Interest in transfusion was revived by the obstetrician James Blundell in 1818. Blundell, faced with uncontrolled fatal puerperal hemorrhage, directed his scientific efforts to the totally neglected operation of blood transfusion. He found the field dominated by antiquated ideas that the blood was "alive." The famous surgeon John Hunter wrote in 1817, "One of the great proofs that the blood possesses life depends upon the circumstances affecting its coagulation. If the blood had not the living principle it would be in respect to the body as an extraneous substance" (Jones and Mackmul 1928).

Blundell devoted himself to perfecting the techniques and devices for the safe and efficient collection of blood for transfusion. He transfused a total of ten patients. Of these, two were already dead, and a third was dying of cancer. His five successes must have been very impressive at the time, and he is properly credited with reviving the use of transfusion and with putting it on a new scientific foundation. Among Blundell's contributions were the concepts that species lines should not be crossed, that it was not necessary to replace all the lost blood, and that small amounts of air injected into the circulation were not necessarily fatal. In addition, he invented a water-jacketed collection funnel and a donor chair similar to those used in modern blood banks (Jones and Mackmul 1928).

When Blundell began his work, the chief potential for blood transfusion was thought to be resurrection. He believed that "death from bleeding (like that of hanging or submersion) may also for a time be apparent . . . it is not impossible that transfusion may be of service within a given time even after breathing has stopped" (Blundell 1824). However, he injected 16 ounces of blood into a woman who had been dead for about six minutes and must have convinced himself that resurrection was an unrealistic goal!

Blundell apparently feared that untoward results might give what he believed to be the erroneous impression that transfusion should be abandoned, and he suggested that adverse cases should not be reported until "a complete body of evidence upon the subject be obtained" (Jones and Mackmul 1928). Of course this proposition was rejected, but his suggestion is very much parallel to today's trend toward not publishing results of experiments with red cell substitutes in the open literature for fear of discouraging progress.

Blundell became embroiled in controversy over his surgical techniques and his revival of the practice of transfusion. He left medical practice after performing only ten transfusions and enjoyed a long retirement. Although there were many attempts to continue Blundell's work, results were sporadic and difficult to understand. Progress was hindered by the lack of understanding of hemolysis, coagulation, and infection. Isolated successes were reported in the literature, but no consistent results could be obtained until these problems were understood.

Coagulation was the first problem to be solved. Bischoff (1835) described the defibrination of blood. By 1875, approximately 347 cases of transfusion were reported in the literature, 129 of which were with animal blood. Apparently only about half of them were successful, and the procedure was reserved for extreme cases, particularly severe hemorrhage (Landois 1875).

After Louis Pasteur had demonstrated that putrefaction was caused by fungi and bacteria, Joseph Lister introduced aseptic techniques in 1867. Thus the two major problems of coagulation and infection were solved over a period of about thirty years.

The remaining problems were not to yield for many more years, and these stimulated a renewed search for a red cell substitute. A brief flurry of interest in transfusion with lamb's blood followed, but a growing awareness of incompatibility prevented its widespread use. In addition, in the period around 1875, physiologic saline was introduced and its safety and efficacy in cases of hemorrhage were demonstrated easily.

The greatest single advance in the use of blood transfusions came in 1900 with the demonstration by Karl Landsteiner (1901) of the presence of isoagglutinating and isoagglutinable substances in the blood. Such substances were shown to be responsible for incompatibility reactions and hemolysis. Many blood groups were described subsequently. The addition of anticoagulants solved another major problem when Hustin (1914) of Belgium reported his experiments using sodium citrate and glucose in the prevention of coagulation. By 1921 the three dangers of heterologous transfusion, incompatibility, infection, and coagulation, were largely controlled. Thus, the need for a red cell substitute decreased again.

1.1.2 World War II

The first modern blood bank was established at the Cook County Hospital in Chicago in 1937 (Diamond 1965), but the first activity in such centers was to store blood plasma for emergency use. There was no organized system for the collection, processing, and distribution of blood and blood products at the outbreak of World War II. Thus the war had a tremendous effect on the blood-banking system and on the use of blood and blood products in the United States. In 1943 Loutit and Mollison, in England, developed a mixture of acid citrate and dextrose which permitted the storage of blood for twenty-one days with a 70 percent viability of cells (Loutit and Mollison 1943). This achievement led directly to the widespread use of blood transfusion on the battlefield and a remarkable lowering of morbidity and mortality.

The American Red Cross collected 13 million units of blood between 1941 and 1945, mainly for processing into dried plasma and later, albumin. The first Allied shipment of blood to the European theater was in August 1944. These units used acid citrate dextrose and were stored up to thirty-eight days. In all, 380,000 units were used in Europe and 180,000 in the Pacific theater.

After the war the many returning physicians and surgeons who had come to rely on these products on the battlefield found they required blood banks and stored blood for their civilian practices. This led to rapid expansion of the blood bank system in the United States. In 1947 the American Red Cross blood banks were established, and by 1963 there were fifty-six of them. In 1948 the American Association of Blood Banks was formed, and the first Red Cross regional blood center was opened in Rochester, New York. By 1976, 10 million units of blood were being collected per year.

1.2 Red Cell Substitutes

The idea of red cell substitutes is not new. In Ovid's *Metamorphosis* the witch Medea restored Jason's aged father, Aeson, by slitting his throat to let out old blood and replacing it with a magic brew she had concocted (Diamond 1980). Sir Christopher Wren was one of the first to apply the new knowledge about the circulation to blood substitutes. In 1656 he infused ale, wine, scammony (a gummy exudate of the plant *Convolvulus scammonia*, a folk-medicine cathartic), and opium into dogs to study their effects. From these efforts, he conceived the idea of transfusing blood from one animal to another as, he claimed, had been suggested to him by the story of Medea and Jason. However, Wren apparently did no more than suggest the possibility of transfusions to Lower, who actually carried out the experiments (Hollingsworth 1928). Wren spent the rest of his long life working in the fields of astronomy and architecture rather than medicine, and he never returned to transfusions or red cell substitutes.

1.2.1 Milk

Milk was one of the first materials to be used as a red cell substitute (Thomas 1878; Jennings 1885; Ringer 1885; Guthrie and Pike 1907; Oberman 1969). Edward Hodder used milk in cases of Asiatic cholera in 1854, and with Thomas he suggested that milk could regenerate white blood cells (Thomas 1878). Two patients were given 12 ounces (or more) of cow's milk and did well, but two others died. In all, Thomas reported twelve cases and concluded that the injection of milk into the circulation in place of blood was a perfectly feasible, safe, and legitimate procedure. These results must have been very exciting, for according to John Brinton (1878), "this new operation will, in a few years, have entirely superseded the transfusion of blood, which latter operation is even now being rejected as at once dangerous and unavailing in many parts of the country."

There were several subsequent reports, and milk was shown to support function in isolated, perfused hearts from a variety of mammals (Guthrie and Pike 1907); however, the transfusion of milk never gained widespread favor and soon disappeared from the literature.

1.2.2 Normal Saline

In the laboratory, the search for a red cell substitute was directed at understanding the physiologic role of blood and its many components rather than at development of clinical applications. *Salzfrosche* were frogs whose blood was completely washed out and replaced with a pure sodium chloride solution. They survived for some hours. "Urea-frogs" and "sugar-frogs" lived longer, but if a small amount of red cells remained, they could survive indefinitely. But frogs are simple animals, and a frog's nervous system can be kept alive for some time without any circulation at all.

1.2.3 Ringer's Lactate

In 1883, Sydney Ringer discovered that the excised ventricle of the frog would beat for some hours if supplied with an aqueous solution of sodium, potassium, and calcium salts. He found that the concentration of potassium and calcium was critical, whereas the amounts of the anions had little effect on the frog heart. The composition of "Ringer's" solution (Table 1.2) was shown many years later to be very close to that of frog plasma. Probably the most popular crystalloid (salt) solution for intravenous use in humans is Ringer's lactate, in which lactate is added to Ringer's solution. The lactate is gradually converted to sodium bicarbonate within the body so that an uncompensated alkalosis is prevented (Hartmann and Senn 1932). But these "crystalloid" solutions cannot support life without red cells; saline passes rather quickly into the tissue spaces of various organs (Miller and Poindexter 1932), especially the liver (Lamson, Robbins, and Greig 1945).

Table 1.2. The Composition of Ringer's Solution

	Ringer's Solution		Frog Plasma
	(g/100 ml)	(mEq/liter)	(mEq/liter)
NaCl	0.6	102	104
KCl	0.0075	1	2.5
$CaCl_2$	0.01	1.8	1.0
$NaHCO_3$	0.01	1.2	25.4

Source: data from Ringer (1885).

1.2.4 Gum-saline

Gum is a galactosidogluconic acid whose molecular mass is approximately 1,500 daltons. First used by Karl Ludwig in kidney perfusion experiments, gum-saline enjoyed great popularity as a plasma expander from the end of World War I onward. However, the aggregation state of gum depends on concentration, pH, salts, and temperature; thus, its colloid osmotic pressure and viscosity are quite variable. Conditions under which the viscosity would be the same as that of whole blood were identified by Bayliss (1920).

In early animal studies, gum was found to coat the surfaces of all blood cells and to promote coagulation. The use of gum-saline became popular in World War I, but it was soon proved not to be efficacious in hemorrhagic shock if the hematocrit was less than 25 percent. In the postwar period, Penfield (1919) showed that gum-saline was less effective than saline alone in treating hemorrhagic shock, but it was useful in stabilizing the blood volume temporarily (Henderson and Haggard 1922). Although throughout the 1920s many reports of anaphylaxis and other untoward reactions appeared, Amberson (1937) claimed that when properly purified, gum-saline was safe for human use. Pharmacologic studies in the 1930s (Amberson 1937) showed that gum was deposited in the liver and spleen and could remain there for many years. Its half-life in the circulation was about thirty hours, and anaphylaxis occurred occasionally. Success with gum-saline became common in the 1930s, but by that time the availability of plasma was such that the need for gum-saline decreased.

1.2.5 Blood Plasma and Serum

The terms *plasma* and *serum* are frequently confused. *Plasma* refers to the liquid that suspends the red cells within the body. *Serum* is that liquid, removed from the body, from which the coagulum has been extracted. This is a very important distinction, because serum contains no coagulation factors and is severely depleted of platelets.

As early as 1871 it was noted that a frog's heart could be maintained by perfusion with sheep and rabbit serum (Bowditch 1871) and that this solution was superior to 0.6 percent NaCl (Kronecker and Stirling 1875). Throughout ensuing years it was recognized that serum exerts a colloid osmotic pressure, contains bicarbonate, and may ensure capillary integrity. Ringer (1885), after dismissing a physiologic role for plasma lipids, eventually agreed that albumin added to a balanced salt solution was superior to the salt solution alone in maintaining the frog's heart.

Claude Bernard recognized that colloids (nondiffusing molecules such as proteins) were important in maintaining water balance. But Ernest Starling (1896) showed clearly that crystalloids (diffusing molecules such as salts) pass through biological membranes easily, whereas colloids do not. Thus, solutions of colloid exert an "oncotic pressure" as water diffuses from the interstitium into vessels, drawn by the imbalance in colloids. In a classic paper, Gilbert Adair (1925b) described in detail the measurement of the colloid osmotic pressure.

In the first half of the present century, much work was devoted to the study of plasma and serum as blood substitutes. One of the problems in this field was the recognition of toxic substances (Moldovan 1910). Reports were published of intravascular coagulation and "vasotonins" that appeared mysteriously after the infusion of serum or plasma. Some workers suggested that this activity could be reduced by heating the serum or by filtering it before use, and some suggested that platelets were to blame. Insulin was implicated by some and adenosine triphosphate (ATP) by others. A major advance in understanding these problems came when the red cell surface antigens were elucidated because the use of serum from donors of blood group AB reduced the vasoconstrictor activity markedly.

By the time Amberson reviewed the field of blood substitutes in 1937, successful exchange transfusions in dogs with either plasma or serum were being demonstrated routinely. The use of plasma in treating massive bleeding was an accepted procedure. Referring to the studies of the toxic effects of plasma and serum, Amberson stated, "We feel that plasma colloids, both protein and fat, probably exercise their major effect by maintaining the colloidal osmotic pressure of blood . . . the normal colloids may be almost completely replaced by other colloids, without injury to the mammalian body, *if there be no oxygen lack.* Oxygen lack undoubtedly occurred in many of the experiments cited above, and the literature is in a state of confusion because of failure to control this and other factors" (Amberson 1937, 54). As we shall see in the following chapters, some of this confusion still exists.

World War II ushered in the modern era of blood fractionation. Owen Wangensteen, at Minnesota, showed that plasma could be administered directly to humans (Wangensteen et al. 1940; Kremen et al. 1942). Although cases of "serum sickness" occurred frequently five to seven days after the infusion, the procedure could be lifesaving in cases of hemorrhagic shock (Dunphy and Gibson 1943).

1.2.6 Albumin

In anticipation of wartime need, the National Research Council asked Edwin J. Cohn, of Harvard University, to investigate the question of whether bovine plasma could be made safe for clinical use. Cohn established an effective multidisciplinary research unit at Harvard, and in 1947 he published the results of their exhaustive studies (Cohn 1947). Using modern protein chemistry methods, including electrophoresis and ultracentrifugation, Cohn showed that most of the adverse reactions were caused by the globulin fraction and that albumin was safe for parenteral use.

1.2.7 Perfluorocarbons

In 1966, Leland Clark and Frank Gollan (1966) demonstrated dramatically that a laboratory mouse could survive total immersion in a perfluorocarbon (PFC) solution (Fig. 1.1). This material, similar to the commercial Teflon, is almost completely inert, but it is also insoluble in water. Henry Sloviter and Kamimoto (1967) prepared a water-soluble emulsion that could be mixed with blood, and Robert Geyer and his colleagues (Geyer, Monroe, and Taylor 1968) were the first to replace completely the blood volume in rats with an emulsion of perfluorotributylamine. The animals survived in an atmosphere of 90–100 percent O_2 and went on to long-term recovery. However, the O_2 content of the PFCs has a linear dependence on PO_2, and a very high O_2 tension is required to transport physiologic amounts of O_2 (Fig. 1.2). This and a propensity to

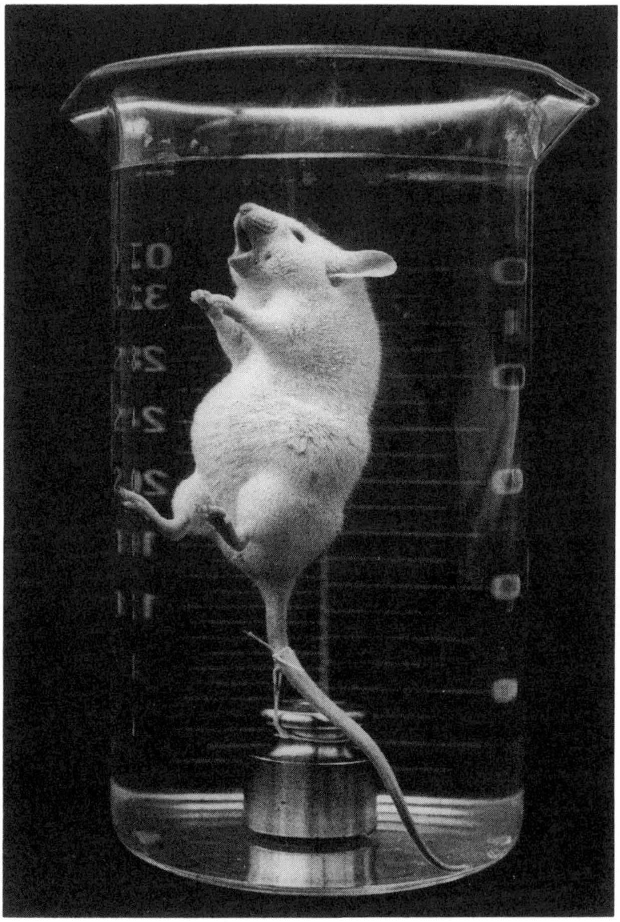

Figure 1.1. Liquid-breathing mouse. The mouse is totally immersed in fluorocarbon (FC - 80, butyltetrahydrofuran), which has been saturated with oxygen by bubbling at room temperature. Such a mouse can survive liquid breathing for many hours. *Source*: Clark (1985), with permission.

be taken up by the reticuloendothelial cells were considered to be severe limitations to the development of clinically useful PFC blood substitutes (Gould et al. 1986a).

Until recently, these problems seemed to present insurmountable hurdles to further development. Now, newer emulsions are being developed which allow higher concentrations of dissolved oxygen, and efforts at developing PFC products are being renewed. One product, Fluosol-DA, a 20 percent (by weight) emulsion, was licensed recently for use in coronary angioplasty, and it is available through the Food and Drug Administration (FDA) for compassionate use.

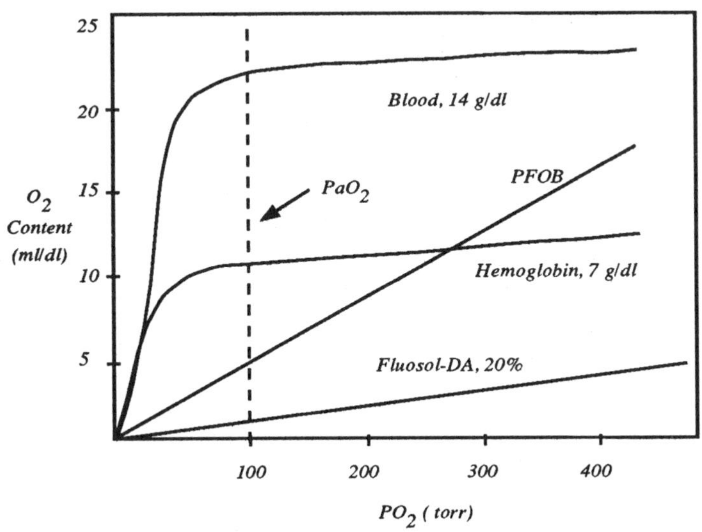

Figure 1.2. Comparison of the oxygen capacity of isooncotic blood (14 g/dl), hemoglobin (7 g/dl), a PFC emulsion (Fluosol-DA, 20%), and perfluorooctalbromide (PFOB). Note that the tetrameric structure of hemoglobin and its cooperativity lead to nearly complete saturation at the arterial oxygen partial pressure, 100 torr.

1.2.8 Cell-free Hemoglobin

Hemoglobin seems to be the logical choice for a red cell substitute because of its high capacity to carry oxygen (Fig.1.2) and its oncotic properties. Probably VonStark (1898) was the first to treat anemic patients with hemoglobin solution. Although his results were encouraging, he was not able to prepare stable solutions and did not pursue the studies further. Better preparations were reported by Sellards and Minot (1916). They administered very small amounts of hemoglobin in an effort to discover its renal threshold and reported no untoward reactions in thirty-three subjects.

Many attempts to administer hemoglobin solutions to humans took place after the reports of Sellards and Minot. But these are difficult to evaluate because the experience was mixed. Many patients did well, but others demonstrated hypertension, bradycardia, oliguria, and even anaphylaxis. These adverse effects were not correlated with specific biochemical properties of the solutions themselves.

1.2.9 Modified Hemoglobin

Although interest in hemoglobin-based red cell substitutes remained extremely high, particularly in wartime, certain difficult problems impaired progress. First, hemoglobin in dilute solution is rapidly cleared by the kidney as the tetrameric protein dissociates into smaller dimers. Second, dilute hemoglobin has a very high affinity for oxygen - so high, in fact, that little of the bound oxygen is released in tissue capillary beds. Third, even exceedingly small amounts of stromal (cell membrane) contaminants in hemoglobin solutions appear to be toxic.

The rapid disappearance of hemoglobin from the circulation was solved when H. Franklin Bunn, working in the U. S. Army Blood Laboratory, discovered that cross-linking with bis(N-maleimidomethyl) ether (BME) prolonged its plasma retention (Bunn and Jandl 1967, 1968b). Bunn and J. H. Jandl concluded that this was because of a reduced tendency to form dimers in the cross-linked hemoglobin, and therefore the hemoglobin was not filtered by the kidney. Accordingly, they showed that most of the hemoglobin could be found in various tissues rather than in the urine.

The problem of the high oxygen affinity of cell-free hemoglobin was solved when Ruth Benesch and Reinhold Benesch discovered reagents that could bind to the 2,3-diphosphoglycerate (2,3-DPG) binding site and reduce the affinity for oxygen (Benesch and Benesch 1967). This discovery led to the description of a variety of modifications of hemoglobin which could not only reduce its oxygen affinity but also stabilize the tetrameric structure so that its vascular retention could be prolonged. The most widely used of these agents is pyridoxal 5'-phosphate (PLP) (Benesch et al. 1972).

In the 1960s many who worked with hemoglobin-based red cell substitutes believed that the contradictory toxicity reports could be explained by contamination of the solutions with foreign materials. S. Frederick Rabiner (Rabiner et al. 1967) studied novel ways to remove stroma from red cell hemolysates and coined the phrase *stroma-free hemoglobin* (SFH). His methods included filtration techniques that could be applied to large volumes of hemolysate and made possible physiologic studies in large animals. Rabiner's results gave new hope to the sagging field because they indicated that the toxic effects of hemoglobin might be prevented by rigorous purification.

After the work of Rabiner and colleagues, several "pure" hemoglobin solutions were produced on a large scale for experimental use. Frank DeVenuto and his colleagues at the Letterman Army Institute of Research described a procedure for "crystallization" of hemoglobin and evaluated the product in a series of animal trials (DeVenuto et al. 1979; DeVenuto, Zegna, and Busse 1979; DeVenuto and Zegna 1981; DeVenuto 1982a, 1982b). The Biotest Serum Institut, Federal Republic of Germany, produced a 6-g/dl hemoglobin solution that had a P_{50} (the PO_2 at which hemoglobin is half-saturated with oxygen) of about 18–20 torr and was used in studies of tissue distribution (Bonhard 1975a). The Warner-Lambert Research Institute in the United States produced a similar solution of SFH which was used for many basic studies of O_2 transport (Biro, Beresford-Kroeger, and Smith 1978) and for a clinical trial in humans (see Chapter 10).

Payne (1973) described protein polymerization with the tissue fixative glutaraldehyde. Soon, a process for polymerizing hemoglobin with the agent was patented by Laver (Laver, Boysen, and Morris 1975), and this material demonstrated a markedly prolonged intravascular retention time. Although the reaction is extremely difficult to control, products for infusion have been developed (Bonhard 1975b; Sehgal et al. 1979; DeVenuto and Zegna 1981). The most successful of these (PLP-polyhemoglobin) is first reacted with PLP and then polymerized with glutaraldehyde; it was the first modified hemoglobin to be used in published human trials (Moss et al. 1989).

Many preparations of modified hemoglobin now have been tested in animals. It appears that most are efficacious in transporting oxygen, and it seems that the more purified the solution, the less its toxicity. The nature of the specific modification appears to affect the biologic properties (e.g., plasma retention time, oxygen affinity, colloid osmotic pressure) more than the toxicity. Several hemoglobin solutions are approaching clinical trials, and it seems possible that within the decade one of them may be available and licensed by the FDA for human use.

Many variations of modified hemoglobin have been studied, including those stabilized with various types of cross-linkers. Some new products are derived from hemoglobin conjugated to synthetic materials such as dextran or polyethylene glycol, and many are well into development as potential red cell substitutes. Sources other than outdated human blood have also been investigated including cow and recombinant hemoglobins produced in bacteria, yeast, and even transgenic mammals.

1.2.10 Encapsulated Hemoglobin

Since hemoglobin is normally packaged inside a membrane, it seems intuitive that encapsulated hemoglobin would be the ultimate solution of the red cell substitute problem. In 1957 Thomas Chang (1988) reported the use of microencapsulated hemoglobin as artificial red blood cells. Since that time, dramatic results have been reported in the complete exchange transfusion of laboratory animals (Djordjevich, Mayoral, and Ivankovich 1985; Hunt et al. 1985), but progress toward development of an artificial red cell for human use has been slow because of problems of reticuloendothelial and other macrophage stimulation (Rabinovici, Rudolph, and Feuerstein 1989). Other problems include maintaining sterility and endotoxin contamination.

1.2.11 Synthetic Heme

Synthetic compounds have been produced which bind or chelate oxygen. These compounds are commercially attractive because their manufacture and licensure may qualify them as drugs, rather than as biologics, with the FDA. Thus, Tsuchida and his colleagues have shown that synthetic hemes can be used to transfuse animals (Tsuchida, Eng, and Nishide 1988). Synthetic oxygen carriers would solve the problem of a limited supply of hemoglobin for modification; at present, however, the synthetic procedures are very tedious, and the possibility of scaleup seems remote.

1.3 Current Status

Several of the products mentioned above are now under intense development. One was approved as an investigational new drug by the FDA, only to have human experimentation halted after unexpected "reactions" in recipients. A second product, based on bovine hemoglobin, was recently approved by the FDA for limited safety testing in humans. Still other hemoglobin-based solutions are also under review at the FDA. Many of the problems described by Amberson have been solved, but others have emerged. This should perhaps not be surprising since replacement of the red blood cells with massive amounts of protein free in solution is an unprecedented therapeutic adventure.

Enthusiasm and despair seem to follow an undulating pattern in this field: progress always seems to reveal new difficulties, and the resulting research always seems to lead to new advances. How long this can be sustained without commercial success is a serious issue because the cost of further development has now outstripped the level of support available from public sources alone.

Chapter 2

Clinical Indications and Properties

2.1 The Impact of Red Cell Substitutes on Transfusion Medicine

Red cell transfusion is big business. More than 13 million units are collected each year in the Unites States alone, and about 10 million units are transfused into 4 million recipients. Of these units, about two-thirds are used during surgery, and the rest are used for either medical or trauma indications. The use of blood and blood products in other parts of the world is not as well known, but represents a significant amount of blood also.

The acquired immune deficiency syndrome (AIDS) epidemic has forced careful attention to the clinical indications for transfusion. All units transfused in the United States in the past five years have been screened for human immunodeficiency virus (HIV), but still about 1 out of 40,000 units can transmit the disease (Busch et al. 1990). Based on 10 million transfusions, this represents a total of about 250 new cases of AIDS per year transmitted by blood that has been screened as HIV negative.

Primarily because of the risk of disease transmission, the number of "frivolous transfusions" is probably now at an acceptably low level (Surgenor et al. 1988). Nevertheless, the supply of red cells in the United States does not meet the demand, and blood is now being imported from Europe. The number of units that outdate is probably less than 5 percent of those collected.

The use of blood, especially type O cells, will continue or increase in the future. A poor cross-match of the major (ABO) blood groups can be accomplished in five to ten minutes, and a better one in fifteen to twenty minutes, but under the best emergency conditions, a complete cross-match still requires about an hour, and it is unlikely that the time can be reduced further. Moreover, clerical and technical errors are more frequent in emergency situations (Goldfinger 1977). Thus, about 200,000 units of type O cells are used in emergency treatment of trauma victims annually.

Continued development of invasive, aggressive medical and surgical procedures will also increase the demands placed on the blood supply. For example, each liver transplantation procedure requires about 100 units of blood (Klein 1989). Furthermore, the increasing mean age of the population will demand more blood and blood products, since the requirement increases with age.

About thirty-five transfusion-related deaths are reported to the Food and Drug Aministration (FDA) each year, most of which are attributed to clerical error (ABO incompatibility) and bacterial infection. Hepatitis-related morbidity and mortality may result from as much as 5 percent of all units transfused (Klein 1989). Although efforts at ridding the blood supply of all viral contamination have been impressive (Chernoff, Klein, and Sherman 1989), no methods of sterilizing cellular components are available currently. It is quite likely that if a sterile, stable, safe alternative to red cells were available, the usage would surely be even higher than the usage of red cells is today.

Table 2.1. Possible Applications for Red Cell Substitutes

Resuscitation after trauma
Elective surgery (hemodilution)
Red cell incompatibility
Ischemic disease and angioplasty
Extracorporeal organ perfusion
Cell culture media
Hematopoietic stimulation
Cardioplegia
Sickle-cell anemia
Tumor therapy
Chronic anemia
Research

The clinical indications for which red cell substitutes would be used are still not defined because the products are not available, and their properties and formulations are not determined. This is important because in any clinical use the benefit of a new agent must be weighed against its risk and against the benefit/risk of existing therapy. Although there appears to be some possibility of HIV transmission by blood screened as negative by immunologic tests (Ward et al. 1988), the risk of transfusion is, in fact, quite low (Zuck 1988; Menitove 1989). Therefore, the burden of proof will be on the developer of any new agent to show that it is as safe and efficacious as current red cell transfusion.

In spite of the lack of products for testing it is nevertheless useful to consider the clinical applications for which these solutions might be developed. This exercise is necessary to plan specific formulations. This chapter will consider a few of the possible applications for hemoglobin-based red cell substitutes (Table 2.1).

2.2 Clinical Indications for Blood Substitutes

2.2.1 Resuscitation after Trauma

One of the most obvious clinical applications for hemoglobin-based red cell substitutes is in emergencies such as trauma. Among the factors that determine the long-term survival after resuscitation from hypovolemic shock is the duration of the shock state (Baker et al. 1985). Messmer and his colleagues (Messmer 1988) have conducted extensive studies of the microcirculation in shock and have pointed out that under the influence of the sympathetic nervous system organ flow is redirected to protect vital organs. Traumatized tissue can be excluded from this control, however, and blood may actually be directed preferentially to sites of bleeding, with consequent hematoma formation. This redistribution of blood flow may protect systemic pressure so that in some instances the degree of shock may not be clinically apparent. Thus, the survival after hemorrhage from severe trauma declines dramatically after the first hour. This critical period has become known as the *golden hour* (Belzberg 1989). Experience during the Korean and Vietnamese conflicts has convinced military physicians that this period is also critical on the battlefield (Mosebar 1989).

The objective of posthemorrhage fluid therapy is to replace lost volume and electrolytes and to reestablish the flow of oxygen to ischemic tissue. This requires restoration of cardiac output as well as tissue reperfusion. Treatment with both colloid and crystalloid (electrolytes) is needed. Available colloids include human serum albumin, dextran, and hydroxyethyl starch. Albumin is not used routinely because of its high cost and short supply. Dextran solutions have antithrombotic properties, but their half-life in the circulation is from two to six hours, and they carry the risk of anaphylaxis.

There can be little doubt that the ideal emergency resuscitation fluid would be one that carries oxygen in addition to providing blood volume expansion. Whole blood or red cells are not routinely used as a first-line resuscitation fluid because of the requirement to cross-match them and because of their high viscosity. Thus, a blood substitute could be aimed at those trauma victims with hypovolemic shock who might otherwise die without immediate restoration of their oxygen supply. Of course, the determination of which patients fall into this category is still problematic.

Since selection of patients for specific parenteral fluid treatment is controversial it is premature to speculate on which would be candidates to receive blood substitutes if they were available. Trauma specialists have disagreed for years on whether crystalloid or colloid is preferred in blood-loss shock (Messmer 1988), but it seems that most patients are eventually given electrolytes, colloids, blood, red cells, and clotting factors at some time during their therapy.

In routine clinical practice, Ringer's lactate is the most widely used primary volume expander. In order to restore the cardiac output with this solution, three to four times the volume of lost blood must be given. Some of this hypooncotic material is lost into the interstitial space, and tissue edema can result. The considerable amounts of oncotically active molecules lost in blood-loss shock must be replaced eventually. Prospective, randomized studies have shown that in fact, hemodynamics were restored faster, with less tissue edema, when dextran 70 was the first fluid used instead of Ringer's acetate (Modig 1983, 1986). Table 2.2 summarizes the current state of the crystalloid versus colloid debate.

Recently, interest in the use of hypertonic-hyperoncotic solutions has been revived. These contain approximately 7.5 g/dl NaCl, usually with a colloid such as dextran 70. A number of investigators have shown that when small volumes of such solutions are given to animals after the induction of hypovolemic shock, the cardiac output is restored almost immediately (Smith et al. 1985; Maningas et al. 1986; Kramer et al. 1986; Kreimeier and Messmer 1987). In addition to the volume expansion properties, lower molecular weight dextran 40 also has antithrombic properties that make it attractive in vascular obstructive disease, hyperviscosity syndromes, and cerebral vascular insufficiency (Messmer 1988; Goslinga 1981).

Hemoglobin solutions have the potential to combine the advantages of crystalloids and colloids. It would seem that most of the desired properties of hypertonic saline-dextran, albumin, and whole blood could be

Table 2.2. Crystalloid versus Colloid Debate.

	Crystalloid	Colloid
Intravascular volume effect		Better
Interstitial volume effect	Better	
Pulmonary edema	Same	Same
Peripheral edema	Common	Rare
Reactions	Uncommon	Occasional
Cost	Inexpensive	Expensive (albumin)
		Moderate (nonalbumin)

Source: Davies (1989), with permission.

combined in a single solution of hemoglobin and electrolytes but with the added advantage of low viscosity. However, the above very brief discussion demonstrates that specification of the properties of this "ideal" solution would be controversial. Add the considerations of oncotic pressure, electrolyte composition and coagulation effects, plasma persistence time, shelf life, and possible toxic effects associated with hemoglobin, and it seems apparent that final formulation of a hemoglobin-containing solution is a long way off, even if a safe solution were available.

The use of type O ("universal") donor cells became widespread during World War II (Camp and Dawson 1974). In the Vietnamese conflict, between 1967 and 1970, 100,419 transfusions were given with only nine reported deaths caused by mismatched blood resulting form clerical error (Camp and Dawson 1974; Camp 1975). By themselves, these figures would not seem to support the development of blood substitutes on the grounds that cross-matching is not necessary. However, if a hemoglobin-based red cell substitute is as useful in the battlefield setting as uncross-matched blood or type O cells then its use could have a tremendous impact on the provision of transfusion services by the military.

Recent military experience in Grenada, Panama, and the Middle East has sugggested that the military requirements for blood could be changing. That is, conflicts now tend to be of high intensity but short duration, placing a potential stress on the blood supply. Hemoglobin-based red cell substitutes could be stockpiled for long periods, presumably, and could be more readily available than whole blood, which requires an elaborate collection, processing, and distribution system.

In the civilian setting, the use of uncross-matched blood or type O cells is much less frequent. In one major center (Yale University) in the years 1974–76, 121 patients received type O cells without further cross-matching (Blumberg and Bove 1978). No untoward effects as a result of the transfusions were noted, and the procedure seemed to have no effect on the overall clinical outcomes. The authors of this study concluded that many of the patients could have been managed with conventional volume expanders and could have waited for proper cross-matching for transfusion. They also pointed out that when uncross-matched blood or type O red cells are available they are used. Clearly, if red cell substitutes devoid of the risks of incompatibility and disease transmission were available, they would be used also.

2.2.2 Elective Surgery

In the United States it is during the perioperative period that most blood and red cells are used. Indications for transfusion have included a hemoglobin concentration less than 10 g/dl (Mollison 1983), but this rule is being reevaluated at present in view of the diminishing blood supply and the recognition of the complications of transfusion (National Institutes of Health Consensus Conference 1988). However, surgical studies suggest that the postoperative period can be shortened and, perhaps, made safer if hemoglobin concentrations are not allowed to fall to less than 10 g/dl.

Although animal studies suggest that the hemoglobin concentration could be reduced safely to about 25 percent of its normal value (Wright 1975), clinical experience suggests that the hemoglobin concentration should not be allowed to drop below 8 g/dl (Carson, et al. 1988). In addition to the prevention of anemia, the outcome of some surgical procedures is improved if blood viscosity can be reduced (Mandel 1986). In these procedures, the combination of low viscosity and maintained oxygen-carrying capacity might optimize transport of oxygen to tissue.

The use of an oxygen-carrying red cell substitute could be invaluable in managing elective surgical procedures. Blood could be collected at the start of the operation and replaced by the oxygen carrier. The removed autologous blood could then be used as needed, either during or after the operation, avoiding the use of homologous blood.

2.2.3 Red Cell Incompatibility

Certain patients develop antibodies to many red cell surface antigens either because they have received multiple transfusions, sometimes over an entire lifetime, or because the existence of unusual antigens has led to minor incompatibilities in the past, with resultant elaboration of antibodies. Some patients simply cannot receive red cell transfusions without undue risk of a fatal reaction. Perhaps blood substitutes could play a role in some of these instances. However, it must be kept in mind that the products being developed now are only oxygen-carrying solutions; they cannot, at present, substitute for other important functions of blood, namely, hemostasis and immunity.

2.2.4 Ischemic Disease and Angioplasty

Tissues that are poorly perfused with blood and therefore receive a marginal supply of oxygen may benefit from increased perfusion with cell-free oxygen carriers. Examples might be ischemic ulcers seen in diabetic or sickle-cell anemia patients and cerebral ischemia. One report (Iwai et al. 1989) demonstrated improved healing of ischemic ulcers when they were bathed in oxygenated perfluorodecalin.

Morbidity during and after percutaneous transluminal coronary angioplasty (PTCA) may be reduced if the myocardium can be perfused with an oxygen carrier. Perfusion with blood is limited because of blood's high viscosity, but perfluorocarbon emulsions have been recently licensed for this application. Solutions of modified hemoglobin with even lower viscosity have been used experimentally (Rossen et al. 1987). This could be a very important application for blood substitutes since a large (and increasing) number of coronary angioplasties is performed in the United States each year. It could also be important for the field of blood substitutes in general because products might be approved more easily for clinical use by the FDA if their indications for use are very circumscribed and if efficacy can be demonstrated easily.

2.2.5 Extracorporeal Organ Perfusion

The preservation of organs for transplantation is an increasing requirement as graft success improves. Hearts, livers, and kidneys might survive better if they could be perfused with an oxygen-carrying solution. Recent work with isolated perfused rabbit hearts has indicated that much more oxygen can be delivered to the myocardium with a hemoglobin-based blood substitute compared with Krebs-Henseleit solution, even if the latter is equilibrated with 100 percent oxygen (Macdonald 1991).

Hemoglobin solutions may be useful in preserving severed limbs for reattachment. Bonhard discussed the use of pyridoxylated hemoglobin in this regard and suggested that postischemia syndrome can be prevented (Bonhard 1988). Steinau and Elert (1980) showed that adenosine triphosphate (ATP) levels were higher and lactate concentrations lower in limbs perfused with hemoglobin solutions rather than with Ringer's lactate.

2.2.6 Cell Culture Media

The recent explosion in cell-cloning technology has increased dramatically the use of cultured mammalian cells for commercial as well as therapeutic and research purposes. It is possible that the quality of these cells and their yield of recombinant gene products can be increased by the use of oxygen-carrying culture media.

2.2.7 Hematopoietic Stimulation

Amberson, Jennings, and Rhode (1949), Hawkins and Johnson (1939), and Gould and colleagues (1988) all noted stimulation of erythropoiesis after administration of cell-free hemoglobin. It is likely that this is a result of the ready availability of heme iron when administered as hemoglobin.

Recombinant human erythropoietin also stimulates red cell production in the preoperative period. Goodnough and his colleagues (Goodnough et al. 1989) showed that 41 percent more autologous blood could be collected from surgical candidates when erythropoietin was administered. Their patients were all given oral iron sulfate during the twenty-one days before surgery. The combined use of erythropoietin and cell-free hemoglobin solution could provide a potent stimulus to endogenous red cell production.

2.2.8 Cardioplegia

During certain surgical procedures such as cardiac valve replacement, repair of congenital anomalies, or aneurysm resection it is necessary to slow or stop the normal heart action. This is done by perfusing the myocardium with various electrolyte solutions and lowering the temperature. Obviously, solutions that transport oxygen to tissues would be desirable since they could both prolong the time allowed the surgeons to operate and speed recovery of function after the procedure.

Elert and Otterman (1979) perfused dog hearts with a solution of pyridoxylated hemoglobin and electrolytes (Table 2.3). They induced cardiac arrest with this solution and measured ATP and phosphocreatine. They were able to show a twenty-minute gain in the time hearts could be stopped, and they had no difficulty in restarting them. On histologic examination, they found less endothelial swelling than in those hearts perfused without hemoglobin.

Table 2.3. Cardioplegia Solution (mEq/liter), pH 7.5

Mg-L-aspartate	5.1
K-DL-aspartate	0.64
Cl^-	14.0
Na^+	38.0
K^+	3.9
$NaHCO_3$	22.0
Procaine hydrochloride	1.10
Glucose monohydrate	2.0
Sorbite	1.40
Polyhemoglobin	64.0

Source: data from Elert and Otterman (1979).

The physiologic requirements for a hemoglobin solution for cardioplegia might be somewhat different from those in other applications. For example the P_{50} should probably be as high as possible (low oxygen affinity) since equilibration of the solution with pure oxygen should be possible, and maximal off-loading at the reduced temperature would be desired. Furthermore, since perfusion of the heart would be local there should be no need to prolong the vascular retention time, and the lowest viscosity possible would be desired. Thus, polymerizaton could be avoided in this application.

2.2.9 Sickle-cell Anemia

Therapy of sickle-cell anemia has a long and controversial history. In this chronic hemolytic anemia, patients "adapt" to a low hemoglobin concentration, and anemia per se is not the main problem. Rather, the rheologic consequences of deformed red blood cells cause morbidity and mortality. The degree of pathologic damage in sickle-cell anemia, moreover, is highly variable from patient to patient, and the clinical course in an individual is completely unpredictable. Some patients may be almost asymptomatic throughout their lives, while others can be severely debilitated. This unpredictability makes the design of clinical trials difficult.

Periodically, sickle-cell patients experience "crisis": episodes characterized by intense pain that can be generalized or localized to specific organs or regions of the body. The pathologic events that underlie these crises involve obstruction of the microvasculature by deoxygenated sickled cells. This obstruction prevents adequate oxygenation of the tissues served by the obstructed capillary beds, and the pain is therefore ischemic.

The red cells of patients with sickle-cell anemia deform ("sickle") when they are deoxygenated, when the pH drops, or when they are dehydrated. When any of these occurs, the viscosity rises dramatically, and circulation slows. Thus, at a given hematocrit, sickle-cell blood has a higher viscosity than normal blood (Charache and Conley 1964).

Oxygen transport can be improved in sickle-cell anemia patients by exchange transfusion with normal red cells (Miller et al. 1980) because a lower viscosity can be achieved without reducing the hemoglobin concentration. Dilution with a hemoglobin solution may be even more effective than exchange transfusion with whole blood. The idea is especially attractive since one of the contraindications to exchange with normal blood is membrane antigen sensitization that eventually occurs after multiple transfusions. In addition, cell-free hemoglobin might be effective in perfusing obstructed capillary beds. In vitro observations suggest that a hemoglobin-polyoxyethylene conjugate may reverse capillary occlusion with sickled cells (Iwasaki et al. 1989).

One difficulty with this application in the United States and Europe is that the sickle-cell patients who are in most need of therapy are those with the poorest venous access; thus, hemodilution with cell-free solutions might still be difficult. An additional limiting factor to this application is that although each individual sickle-cell patient is very dependent on the health care system, the total number of patients may not justify the development of commercial products. In African countries, however, where the incidence of sickle-cell anemia is much higher, these products could have a major impact on health care. In these countries the risk of transmission of HIV by blood transfusion is extremely high.

2.2.10 Tumor Therapy

Some treatments of soft tissue tumors involve local destruction of malignant tissue by activated oxygen. Thus, any method for increasing tissue oxygen tension could be viewed as an adjunct. The perfluorocarbons have been suggested for this application, but if proven safe, hemoglobin could also be useful for some types of therapy. In this case, the optimal product would have the highest P_{50} possible since the solution would be oxygenated outside of the body and infused directly into the circulation of the tumor.

An alternative approach has already been shown to be effective in animals. Drugs (clofibrate, bezafibrate, and gemfibrozil) that reduce oxygen affinity dramatically (rise of from 10 to 20 torr in the P_{50} value) were administered to tumor-bearing mice. Marked sensitization to irradiation was observed when these animals were given supplemental oxygen to breathe (Hirst, Wood, and Schwartz 1987).

If a high "arterial" oxygen tension is achievable, then perfluorocarbons might be the perfusion medium of choice since photoactivation of heme-containing drugs also could be used (hemoglobin would absorb much of the delivered light energy). These applications could be fairly widespread, eventually, and commercialization might be attractive since the volume of agent would be much less than in high-volume resuscitation or hemodilution applications.

2.2.11 Chronic Anemia

Chronic anemia would *not* seem to be a good indication for blood substitutes. First, patients usually adapt to chronic anemia just as high-altitude natives seem to become acclimatized to chronic hypoxia. The inability of the currently developed blood substitutes to provide coagulation factors, platelets, or leukocytes would not seem to be a major drawback, especially in patients with chronic hemolysis, red cell aplasia, cancer, or other types of chronic disease.

If a red cell substitute were developed for chronic anemia it would need to have the longest possible plasma retention to eliminate the need for excessively frequent infusions. The products that might be candidates to fill this need would be encapsulated or conjugated hemoglobin or derivatives with a very high molecular weight. Most efforts have been directed toward development of perfluorocarbons with short retention times and of hemoglobin solutions with intermediate times.

2.2.12 Research

Sixteen years ago, Geyer (1975) reviewed the potential uses of blood substitutes. The list of anticipated clinical applications was much like the one above and was the driving force behind commercialization and therefore availability of products. But Geyer also listed prominently a number of research areas that will benefit from the availability of these products. They will be extremely useful in basic studies of hematopoiesis, protein metabolism, all aspects of oxygen transport, including the microcirculation, and utilization of oxygen by tissues, and particularly the differences between specific organs. This research will not only advance basic knowledge of biochemistry and physiology but will doubtless give rise to new clinical uses that are not appreciated now.

2.3 Requirements for a Blood Substitute

Some of the required properties of red cell substitutes are obvious. They must be sterile, free of endotoxin and viruses, nontoxic, and efficacious, and it must be possible to store them for reasonable periods. The methods used to produce them must be tractable for industrial scaleup and not too expensive. Lot-to-lot variation and immunogenicity must be minimal.

These requirements can pose serious industrial problems, particularly when large batches must be prepared in a routine fashion. Some of the other properties would be tailored to the individual products under development, and their specifications are more controversial (see Table 2.4).

It is clear that the properties of a hemoglobin solution intended for parenteral use should be matched to the clinical indication. For example, administration in a case of chronic, refractory anemia would require a long plasma retention and normal colloid osmotic pressure. A solution for resuscitation from acute blood loss should have an increased colloid osmotic pressure but short plasma retention because blood would be available to the patient within several hours of injury in most cases. The patient who is unable to maintain a normal alveolar oxygen tension might do better with a reduced P_{50}, but when arterial oxygen tension can be elevated a high P_{50} would favor tissue oxygen delivery. In some applications, such as organ preservation for transplantation, the properties are probably less critical because more control of oxygenation and temperature, for example, is possible.

Table 2.4. Physiologic Properties for Various Clinical Applications

Application	P_{50}	COP	$t_{1/2}$
Resuscitation (military)	nl[a]	High	6–10 h
Resuscitation (civilian)	nl	High	20–30 h
Hemodilution	High	nl	10–20 h
Erythropoiesis	nl	nl	Short
Organ preservation	nl	nl	Irrelevant
Angioplasty	nl	nl	Short?
Anemia	nl	nl	Maximal
Sickle-cell anemia	nl	High?	Short
Tumor therapy	High	nl	Short
Cell culture	nl	nl	Irrelevant

[a] *nl*: normal; as usually found in humans.

2.3.1 Oxygen Capacity

A red cell substitute must, of course, carry oxygen, but it is difficult to specify how much. Perhaps the oxygen-carrying capacity of blood with a normal hemoglobin concentration is not necessary, but there are no guidelines as to the minimal hemoglobin concentration required for health. For years surgeons and anesthesiologists have used the "10 - gram rule" in the belief that a hemoglobin concentration less than 10 g/dl will impair tissue healing. As pointed out earlier, perhaps this figure can be safely dropped to 8 g/dl.

2.3.2 Oxygen Affinity

Another difficult specification is the oxygen affinity of the prospective red cell substitute. As a first approximation, it would seem logical that the P_{50} should be that of normal human blood, but it is known that even in natives of high altitude, variation around the normal P_{50} of about 28 torr does not seem to affect oxygen transport (Winslow and Monge 1987).

Although the determination of the lowest and highest values for P_{50} is approximate at best, some rough limits can be set. Abnormal human hemoglobins with P_{50} values in the area of 19 torr lead to polycythemia, showing that oxygen delivery to the renal site of erythropoietin production in these cases is compromised. The upper boundary for the acceptable P_{50} is much more controversial. Some workers believe that there is no limit to the benefit of increased P_{50}, but this depends on the ability of the lung to oxygenate blood. That is, if 100 percent saturation is reached in the lung, it is likely that the higher the P_{50}, the more easily oxygen can be unloaded in the tissues. This would be the case in a patient undergoing elective surgery in which arterial oxygen tension is controlled. However, if pulmonary oxygenation is compromised in any way, the uptake in the lung becomes an issue, and a lower P_{50}, rather than higher, is beneficial (Winslow, Samaja, and West 1984). A high P_{50} would also be desired in tumor therapy to maximize tissue oxygen tension.

Less obvious than these considerations is the importance of the Bohr effect, cooperativity, and carbon dioxide transport. In the absence of better guidelines, it seems reasonable that a red cell substitute should bind oxygen cooperatively, should exhibit a Bohr effect, and should transport carbon dioxide. It should be noted that only one relevant study of carbon dioxide transport in a potential red cell substitute has been reported (Vandegriff et al. 1991).

2.3.3 Viscosity

The viscosity of a blood substitute is a critical issue, since the bulk viscosity of whole blood is an exponential function of hematocrit (Fig. 2.1). Some workers have reported that oxygen delivery to the brain may be compromised when the hematocrit is elevated even to the high-normal range (Humphrey et al. 1979). At equivalent hemoglobin concentrations,

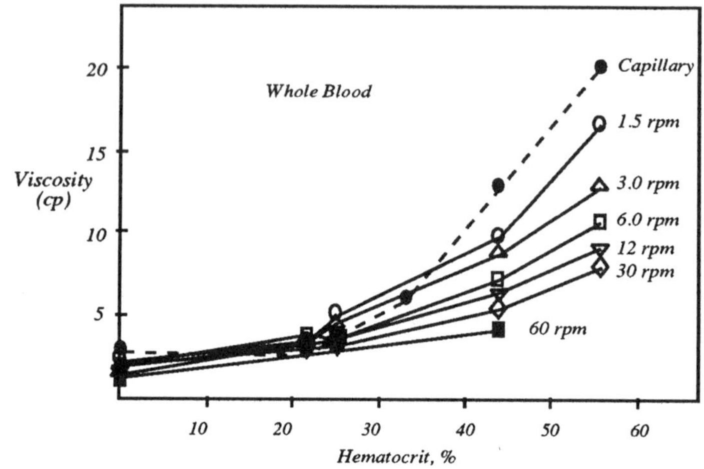

Figure 2.1. Dependence of viscosity of whole blood on hematocrit. Viscosity measurements were made using a rotating cone-and-plate viscometer at different shear rates. The curve labeled *capillary* represents measurements made in a capillary viscometer designed to simulate very low-flow capillary beds.

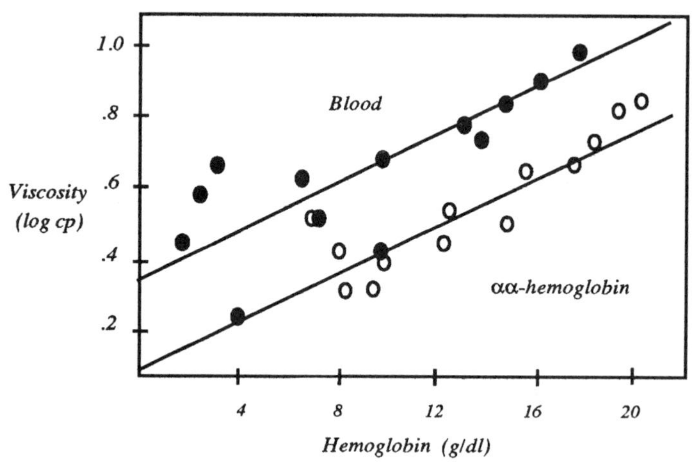

Figure 2.2. Comparison of blood and αα-hemoglobin viscosity, measured at 3 rpm in a rotating cone-and-plate viscometer. Note that at a given viscosity, the concentration (and therefore O_2 capacity) of the αα-hemoglobin solution is about 8 g/dl higher than for whole blood.

cross-linked hemoglobin has a lower viscosity than whole blood at the low shear rates found in capillaries (Fig. 2.2). When the blood substitute is polymerized hemoglobin, the viscosity increases with the degree of polymerization. Thus, there is some theoretical basis for the belief that the lowest possible viscosity is desirable.

Red cell suspensions are non-Newtonian in their flow patterns; that is, in vivo flow is turbulent, and red cells stream. These two properties are dependent on the diameter of the vessel. Turbulence is probably important to red cell oxygen transport because of stirring in the area immediately surrounding the cell. In contrast, cell-free hemoglobin solutions will be homogeneous with respect to flow. The effect on oxygen delivery in tissue capillary beds is unpredictable.

2.3.4 Plasma Retention

A red cell substitute must have a reasonable intravascular persistence. Although the length of time the oxygen carrier should remain in the circulation is not defined clearly (Greenburg et al. 1982), a period of twenty to forty hours is often cited. Vagueness in this specification is not surprising since the clinical indications for such solutions have not been determined. Additional considerations are the toxicity and route of removal from the circulation. Modified hemoglobins are not removed primarily by renal mechanisms (Keipert and Triner 1989); rather, these materials are taken up by the macrophage-monocyte (reticuloendothelial) system and other tissues. If the solutions are toxic, then the least possible exposure would seem desirable, and they should be used only in emergency situations, probably for resuscitation. If the solutions are not toxic, then a longer intravascular persistence would seem permissible, and a wider clinical application might be established.

The polymerized hemoglobin products and hemoglobin conjugated to dextran or other polymers have the longest intravascular retention times. Hemoglobins cross-linked at intramolecular sites all seem to have retention times prolonged three to five times longer than unmodified hemoglobin, but the actual times are species and dose dependent (Hess et al. 1989, Fig. 2.3). The retention in humans will not be known until appropriate clinical trials are performed, and doses can be administered which are higher than those used in the limited safety trials carried out to date.

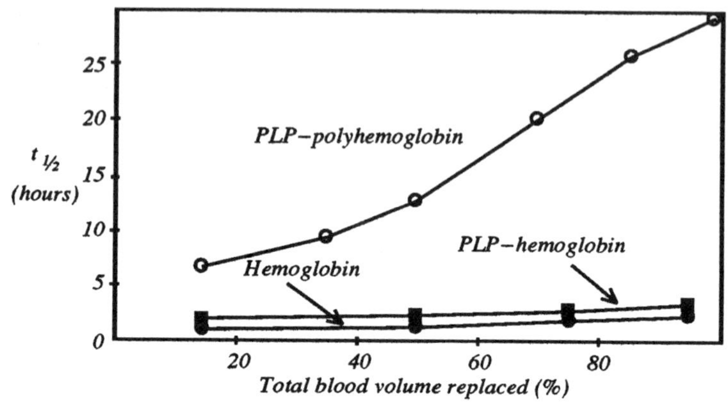

Figure 2.3. Plasma retention ($t_{1/2}$) of injected hemoglobin in the circulation as a function of the percentage of blood volume replacement. *PLP*, pyridoxal 5'-phosphate. *Source*: Keipert and Chang (1987), with permission.

2.3.5 Colloid Osmotic Pressure

It is important to emphasize the fundamental differences between solutions that exert a colloid osmotic pressure (colloids) and those that exert only an osmotic pressure (crystalloids). Colloid solutions are those that contain particles that are osmotically active but which do not diffuse across biologic membranes. Crystalloids are also osmotically active, but the molecules can diffuse across membranes. Thus, both solutions expand the intravascular space immediately, but the effect of colloid solutions persists longer.

One of the chief arguments for the polymerization of hemoglobin has been that when the molecular weight is increased the concentration of molecules is less even though the oxygen carried is the same (Fig. 2.4). Thus, pyridoxylated, polymerized hemoglobin can be infused into animals to achieve a final concentration of 15 g/dl and a normal colloid osmotic pressure. In this case, there are no major shifts of water between the interstitial and intravascular spaces. In contrast, unpolymerized hemoglobin with a molecular mass of 64,000 daltons has increased colloid osmotic pressure; only about 7 g/dl can be achieved because infusion requires a shift of water from the interstitium into the intravascular space to maintain oncotic balance (Hess et al. 1989). Some workers in the trauma

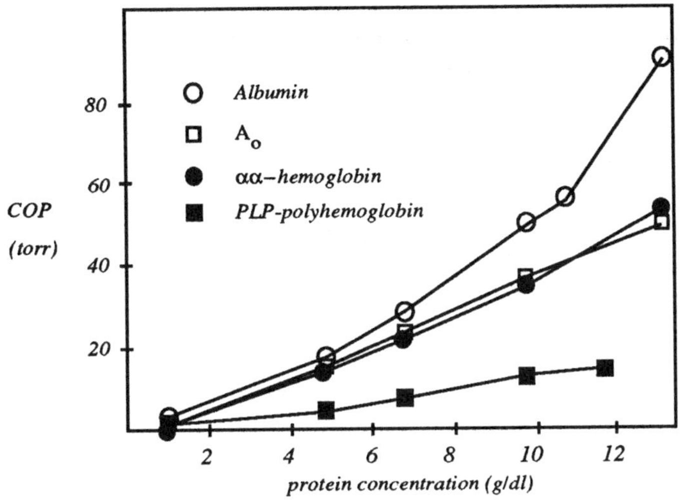

Figure 2.4. Colloid osmotic pressure (*COP*) of hemoglobin solutions as a function of protein concentration. Note that at a given concentration, the higher molecular mass materials such as polymerized hemoglobin (PLP-polyhemoglobin) have a lower COP than hemoglobin cross-linked between α chains (αα-hemoglobin), unmodified hemoglobin (A_o), or albumin. *PLP*, pyridoxal 5'-phosphate.

field believe hyperoncotic solutions are preferred for resuscitation because volume expansion can be achieved more rapidly than with the infusion of large quantities of isotonic solutions. Menu et al. (1985) actually showed improved survival in rats with cell-free hemoglobin when the concentration was 12.5 g/dl rather than 7.0 g/dl despite (or maybe because of) a very high colloid osmotic pressure.

2.3.6 Storage Stability

Obviously, storage stability is an extremely important property for any blood substitute. The longer the product can be stored, the more cost effective it will be. Since there are no products yet available for clinical use, it is not possible to evaluate their stability. Lyophilization is feasible (Greenburg, Ginsburg, and Peskin 1977; DeVenuto, Zegna, and Busse 1979) although the temperature of storage is important.

The main deterioration of stored hemoglobin will be its oxidation to methemoglobin. This reaction is complex, and its rate will depend on the specific chemical modification, the ionic environment, the formulation, and the environmental conditions. Oxidation reactions in normal human hemoglobin are still not understood completely, so such studies will be necessarily empirical in the near future. However, is it possible that by the systematic study of oxidation mechanisms in a variety of modified and mutant hemoglobins, new insights into the reaction will be achieved.

Chapter 3

The Structure and Function of Hemoglobin

Hemoglobin is a globular protein whose molecular mass is about 64,000 daltons. It is composed of four subunit polypeptide chains (globin) of about 140 amino acids each. Each chain has a molecular mass of 16,100 daltons and carries a tetrapyrrole iron-containing prosthetic group, heme, which can bind one molecule of oxygen. In humans several hemoglobins occur normally, but all contain four subunits: the differences are limited to the primary structure (amino acid sequence) of globin.

Each polypeptide chain is designated by a Greek letter, and each is the product of a specific gene. For example, hemoglobin A, the major component of adult human red blood cells, is $\alpha_2\beta_2$; that is, it contains two α chains and two β chains in a tetrameric arrangement. The normally occurring hemoglobins in humans and their polypeptide components are shown in Table 3.1. In addition to these hemoglobins, human red cells also contain variable amounts of glycosylated hemoglobins, such as hemoglobin A_{1c}.

Table 3.1. The Hemoglobins of Adult Human Red Cells

A_o	$\alpha_2\beta_2$	Main component of human red cells
F	$\alpha_2\gamma_2$	Fetal hemoglobin
A_2	$\alpha_2\delta_2$	Minor component of human red cells
	$\alpha_2\zeta_2$	Embryonic hemoglobin

3.1 Structure

3.1.1 Primary structure

Hemoglobin was one of the first proteins whose primary structure (sequence) was determined (Fig. 3.1). Today, elucidation of a sequence which would have taken years three decades ago is a relatively trivial matter. The high-resolution X-ray crystallographic analysis by Perutz and co-workers (Bolton and Perutz 1970) allowed an extensive integration of sequence and functional data. This integration leads to an appreciation of structure-function relationships so delicate that substitution of one amino acid in 280 can lead to serious clinical consequences, as in sickle-cell anemia. It is not surprising that when hemoglobin is modified chemically in the production of red cell substitutes, significant alterations in function can be expected, and these must be understood before toxicity and efficacy trials can be interpreted.

3.1.2 Secondary Structure

About two-thirds of the residues of each chain are arranged in seven and eight helices of the α and β chains, respectively (see Fig. 3.2). The helices are designated from A to H, and vary from seven to twenty residues in length. There are 3.6 residues per turn of helix, which are stabilized by hydrogen bonds formed longitudinally along their axes. The remaining one-third of the residues is distributed over corners or nonhelical regions of the chain.

Myoglobin and all the various hemoglobin chains resemble each other to a remarkable degree. To emphasize this resemblance and to facilitate comparison among chains, residues are given designations according to their position in or between helical regions. For example, residue 10 of the α chain is valine A7(10)α because it occupies position 7 from the beginning of the A helix. Although the corresponding residue in the β chain is valine A7(11)β, it occupies the eleventh position from the amino terminus of that chain. Similarly, the residues in the interhelical regions are given designations using letters of adjacent helices: the third residue in the C-D region of the α chain, for example, is histidine CD3(45)α, and in the β chain, serine CD3(44)β.

					A							
α	Val	-	Leu	Ser	Pro	Ala	Asp	Lys	Thr	Asn	Val	Lys
β	Val	His	Leu	Thr	Pro	Glu	Glu	Lys	Ser	Ala	Val	Thr
							A		B			
α	Ala	Ala	Try	Gly	Lys	Val	Gly	Ala	His	Ala	Gly	Glu
β	Ala	Leu	Try	Gly	Lys	Val	Asn	Val	-	-	Asp	Glu
α	Tyr	Gly	Ala	Glu	Ala	Leu	Glu	Arg	Met	Phe	Leu	Ser
β	Val	Gly	Gly	Glu	Ala	Leu	Gly	Arg	Leu	Leu	Val	Val
	C											
α	Phe	Pro	Thr	Thr	Lys	Thr	Phe	Pro	His	Phe	-	Asp
β	Tyr	Pro	Try	Thr	Gln	Arg	Phe	Glu	Ser	Phe	Gly	Asp
			D							E		
α	Leu	Ser	His	Gly	Ser	Ala	-	-	-	-	-	Gln
β	Leu	Ser	Thr	Pro	Asp	Ala	Val	Met	Gly	Asn	Pro	Lys
α	Val	Lys	Gly	His	Gly	Lys	Lys	Val	Ala	Asp	Ala	Leu
β	Val	Lys	Ala	His	Gly	Lys	Lys	Val	Leu	Gly	Ala	Phe
α	Thr	Asn	Ala	Val	Ala	His	Val	Asp	Asp	Met	Pro	Asn
β	Ser	Asp	Gly	Leu	Ala	His	Leu	Asp	Asn	Leu	Lys	Gly
		F										
α	Ala	Leu	Ser	Ala	Leu	Ser	Asp	Leu	His	Ala	His	Lys
β	Thr	Phe	Ala	Thr	Leu	Ser	Glu	Leu	His	Cys	Asp	Lys
				G								
α	Leu	Arg	Val	Asp	Pro	Val	Asn	Phe	Lys	Leu	Leu	Ser
β	Leu	His	Val	Asp	Pro	Glu	Asn	Phe	Arg	Leu	Leu	Gly
α	His	Cys	Leu	Leu	Val	Thr	Leu	Ala	Ala	His	Leu	Pro
β	Asn	Val	Leu	Val	Cys	Val	Leu	Ala	His	His	Phe	Gly
				H								
α	Ala	Glu	Phe	Thr	Pro	Ala	Val	His	Ala	Ser	Leu	Asp
β	Lys	Glu	Phe	Thr	Pro	Pro	Val	Gln	Ala	Ala	Tyr	Gln
α	Lys	Phe	Leu	Ala	Ser	Val	Ser	Thr	Val	Leu	Thr	Ser
β	Lys	Val	Val	Ala	Gly	Val	Ala	Asn	Ala	Leu	Ala	His
α	Lys	Tyr	Arg									
β	Lys	Tyr	His									

Figure 3.1. The primary structure (amino acid sequences) of the α and β polypeptide chains of adult human hemoglobin. Helical regions are designated by *letters A* to *H* and are shaded. *Source*: adapted from Morimoto, Lehmann, and Perutz (1971).

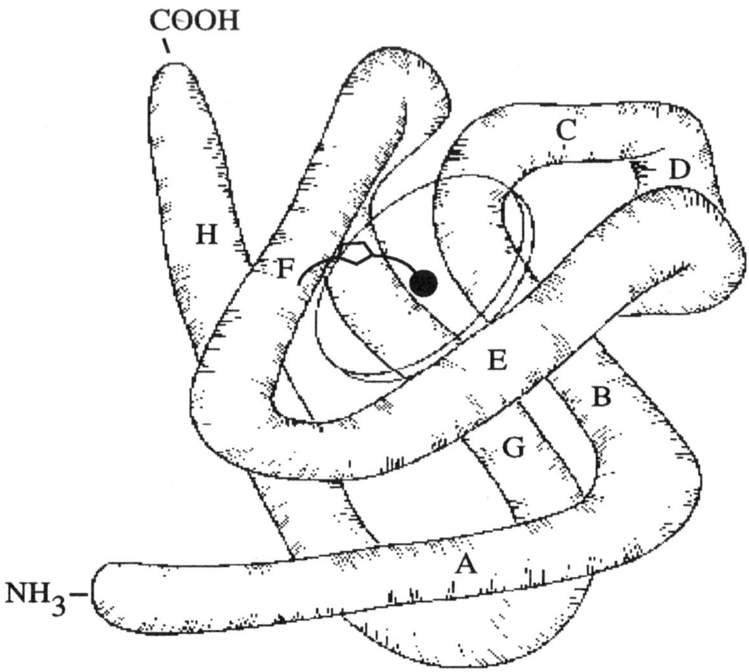

Figure 3.2. Schematic diagram of a globin chain. Any of the globin chains could fit the diagram with only minor alterations. The α-helical regions are *lettered* (compare Fig. 3.1). The heme is shown as a *disc*. The only covalent link between heme and globin is between the iron atom and histidine F8, the proximal histidine.

3.1.3 Tertiary Structure

The three-dimensional folding of a globin chain is also shown in Figure 3.2. The similarity among the various chains is sufficient so that the figure could represent any of them with only minor alterations. Heme is represented as a flat ring between the E and F helices.

Proline does not fit into a helix because of its pyrrolidine ring; it cannot form hydrogen bonds with the next coil in the helix. Therefore, it is likely to occur at corners and interhelical regions. Other corners are stabilized by a variety of stereochemical mechanisms, some of which involve portions of chains that lie nearby. Interactions can also occur between helical segments that lie in proximity to one another. For example, the B and E helices are stabilized in each helix by glycine residues, which afford a compact fit at their crossing.

A very important force stabilizing the globin chain structure is the presence of heme itself. Free globin is much less soluble than the molecule containing heme. It is embedded firmly into a "pocket" in the chain as shown in Figure 3.2. It has polar and nonpolar ends, one formed by propionic acid groups and the other by vinyl and methyl groups, respectively. The amino acid side groups lining the heme pocket are largely nonpolar and allow the heme to enter, vinyl end first. It is then anchored there by a large number of interactions between the pyrrole ring and amino acids of the heme pocket. In addition, it is linked covalently to histidine F8, which is called the *proximal* histidine. The *distal* histidine E7 is not linked covalently to the heme group, but its presence in the heme pocket is important in maintaining spatial relationships. The hydrophobic nature of the heme pocket is extremely important in the maintenance of the heme iron in its reduced (Fe^{2+}) state, which is required for oxygenation. A number of mutations in the environment of the heme pocket can lead to the entry of water, oxidation of the iron, and as a result, methemoglobin formation.

New details about the molecular mechanism of ligand binding in the heme pocket have been revealed by the study of site-directed mutants. Perutz proposed that the distal histidine (E7) acts as a "gate" to allow ligand to enter the heme pocket only when it swings out (Perutz 1989). In the α chain (or myoglobin), a hydrogen bond forms between N_ε of histidine E7 and the oxygen molecule (Fig. 3.3).

When histidine E7 is replaced by glycine in site-specific mutants, free access to the heme pocket is permitted. The result is that oxygen affinity and kinetic constants are unchanged for the R-state β chain, but the oxygen affinity is reduced fourteenfold in R-state myoglobin and eightfold in α chains (Olson et al. 1988). This is interpreted to mean that the rate of movement of histidine E7(63)β is so fast as to not restrict entry of ligand into the heme pocket. In contrast, the stabilization of oxygen by histidine E7(57)α accounts for the relatively higher affinity for oxygen by the α chain relative to the β chain.

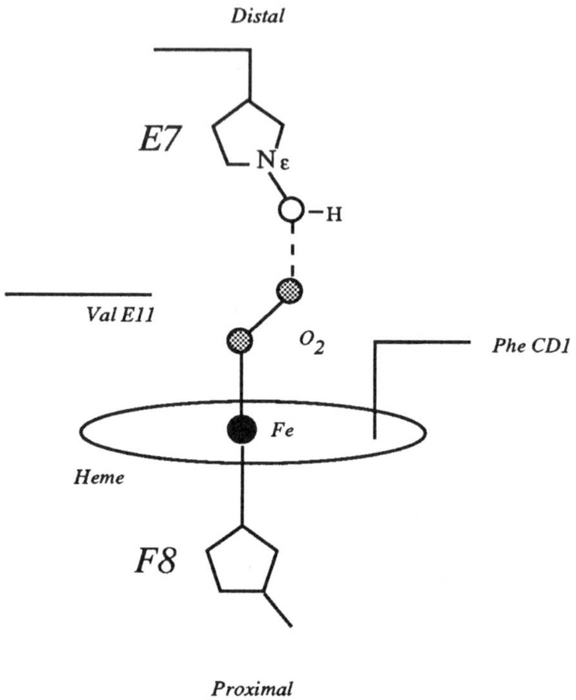

Figure 3.3. Arrangement of the proximal and distal residues in myoglobin, showing the bonds that stabilize oxygen in the heme pocket. Histidine E7 acts as a gate to permit or restrict entry of the oxygen molecule into the pocket. *Source*: adapted from Perutz (1989).

3.1.4 Quaternary Structure

The association of globin chains into a tetrameric structure (Fig. 3.4) leads to cooperativity, the Bohr effect, the 2,3-diphosphoglycerate (2,3-DPG) effect, and suitable oxygen affinity so that tissue oxygen requirements can be met. The molecule has a twofold axis of symmetry, each half containing one α and one β chain, which are held tightly together by a large number of atomic interactions. There are four areas of contact between the subunits: $\alpha_1\beta_1$, $\alpha_2\beta_2$, $\alpha_2\beta_1$, and $\alpha_1\beta_2$. The $\alpha_1\beta_2$ and $\alpha_2\beta_1$ regions are somewhat weaker than the $\alpha_1\beta_1$ and $\alpha_2\beta_2$ contacts and allow movement during oxygenation (Fig. 3.5).

Isolated hemoglobin chains are less stable than the fully associated tetramers. Thus, the regions of contact between them are important in maintaining normal solubility. Several unstable mutants involve the $\alpha_1\beta_1$ and, to a lesser degree, the $\alpha_1\beta_2$ contacts.

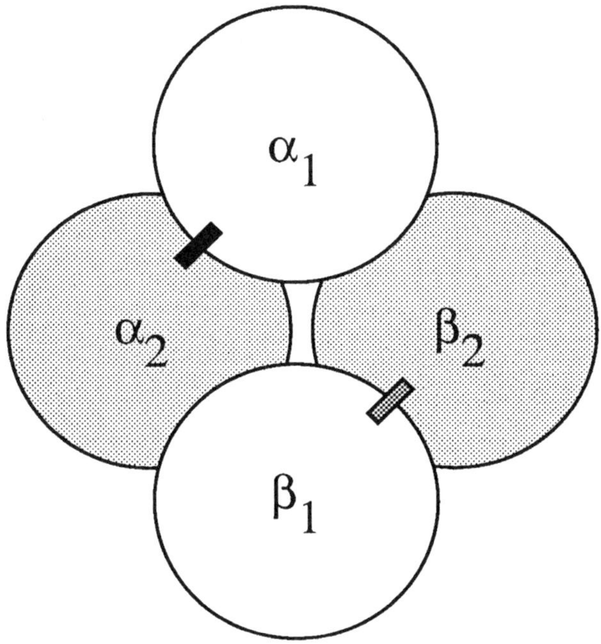

Figure 3.4. The quaternary structure of hemoglobin. αβ subunits are shown as either shaded or plain. The subunits are held together by many interactions at the interfaces, but inside the red cell 2,3-DPG (stippled rectangle) reduces dissociation. Chemical cross-linking, for example with bis(3,5-dibromosalicyl)fumarate (DBBF, filled rectangle) between α chains, also stabilizes the molecule.

The central cavity of hemoglobin is filled with water and allows the entrance of charged molecules that affect molecular function, such as 2,3-DPG and salts. Most of the charged amino acid side groups are directed toward the outside of the molecule and enter into electrostatic relations with solvents, allowing very high solubility within the red blood cells. Buried in the midst of the globin chains are the four heme groups containing ferrous iron, protected against oxidation by a hydrophobic environment.

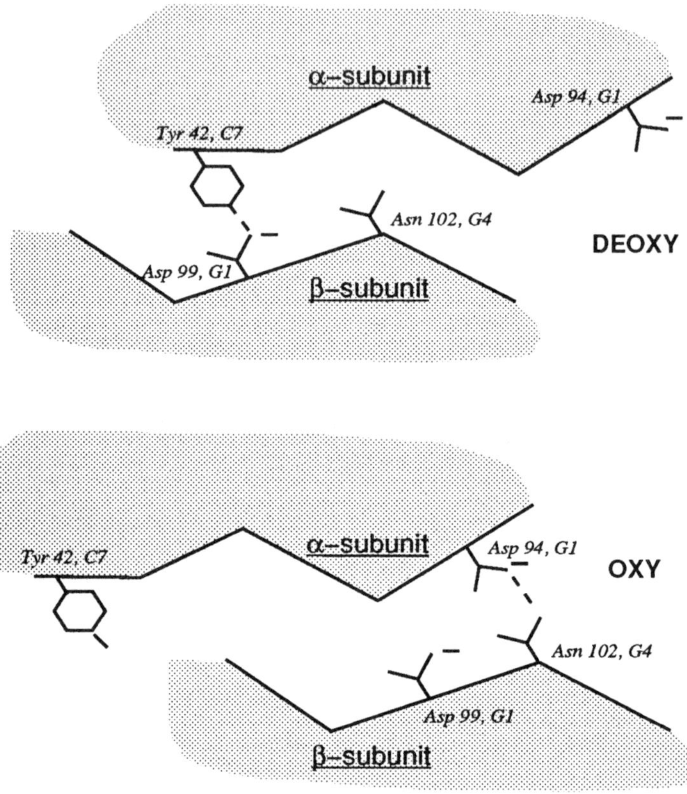

Figure 3.5. Changes at the $\alpha_1\beta_2$ interface on oxygenation. The contact "clicks" from one dovetailed structure to another, involving a switch from one hydrogen bond to a second. The other bonds are nonpolar. *Source:* adapted from Morimoto, Lehman, and Perutz (1971).

3.1.5 Two Quaternary Conformations

The function of hemoglobin in oxygen binding can best be understood on the basis of at least two separate quaternary conformations, corresponding to the oxy and deoxy states. Perutz and his associates described these two structures using X-ray crystallography and related them to the R (for relaxed) and T (for tense) conformations (Bolton and Perutz, 1970). They found that the combination of deoxyhemoglobin with oxy-

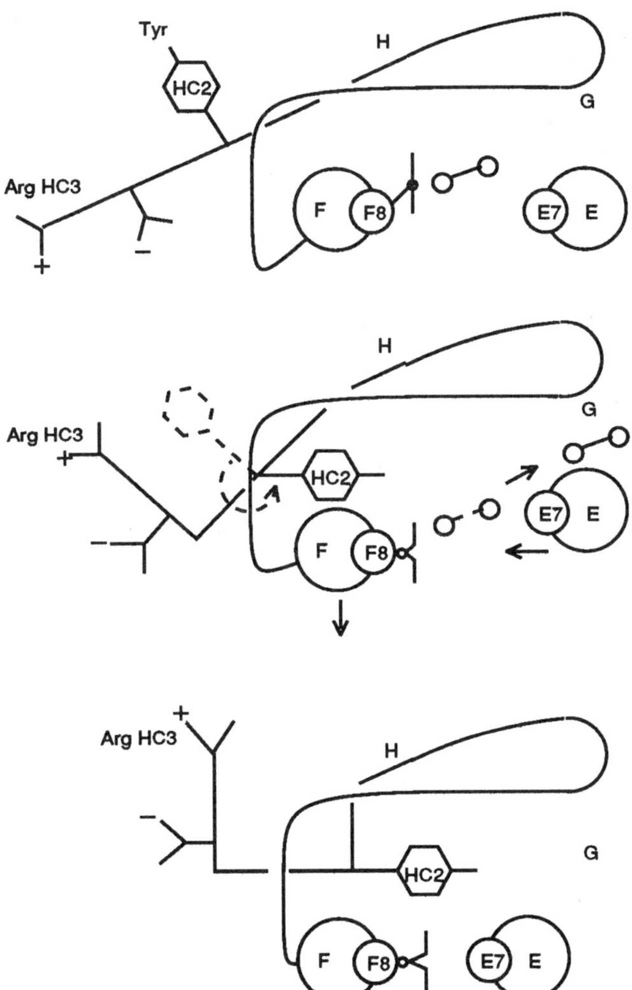

Figure 3.6. The changes in the tertiary structure of hemoglobin produced by the transition from the oxy (top) to deoxy (bottom) conformations. When oxygen moves out of the heme pocket, the E helix moves into and the F helix moves out of the heme pocket, providing a space for the phenolic group of tyrosine HC2. Arginine HC3 is pulled into position to form salt bridges. *Source:* adapted from Charache (1974).

gen produced shifts of the helical regions of 2 to 3 Å, and a change in the tilt of the heme group relative to the globin chain. This is accompanied by shifts of the iron atom within the porphyrin and of the heme-linked histidine (Fig. 3.6).

In the deoxy β subunit the γ-methyl group of valine E11(67) blocks the heme pocket. In the oxy form (R) this pocket widens, making room for the binding of an oxygen molecule. There is little difference at the $\alpha_1\beta_1$ (and $\alpha_2\beta_2$) contact, but a significant change at the $\alpha_1\beta_2$ (and $\alpha_2\beta_1$) contact occurs. The region is dovetailed so that the CDα region of one chain fits into the FGβ region of the other. During transition from R to T, the dovetailing between CDα and FGβ changes so that the hydrogen bond linking aspartate G1(94)α to asparagine G4(102)β is replaced by another between tyrosine C7(42)α and aspartate G1(99)β (Fig. 3.5).

Finally, large differences occur in the areas of the carboxyl-terminal residues. In deoxyhemoglobin the tyrosines (HC2) occupy pockets between helices F and H, and their phenolic groups are hydrogen bonded to valines FG5. The carboxyl-terminal residues are constrained by participation in salt bridges (Fig. 3.7). In oxyhemoglobin, the phenolic groups of tyrosine HC2α are ejected from their pockets, and the salt bridges are broken.

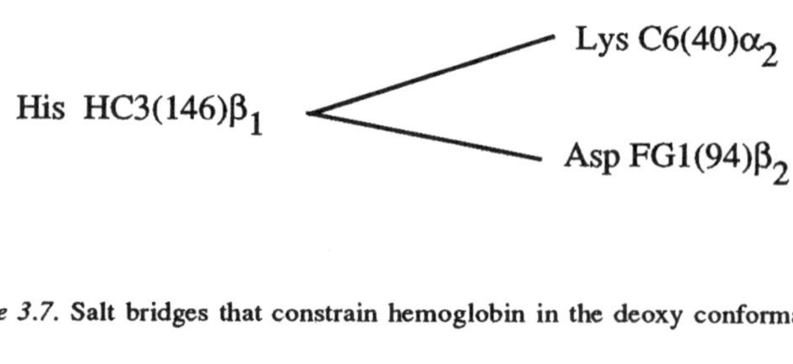

Figure 3.7. Salt bridges that constrain hemoglobin in the deoxy conformation.

Perutz and co-workers proposed a model that relates these molecular changes to oxygen binding. The first, or *trigger*, step results from the combination of iron with oxygen. When this occurs, the atomic radius of iron decreases (high-to-low spin transition), allowing it to move closer to the plane of the porphyrin ring. This movement is less than 1 Å, but it is sufficient to change the distance between the heme-linked histidine and the plane of the porphyrin ring, initiating the sequence of changes leading to the T to R transition. This description applies to the α chain; but in β, the hydrophobic side group of valine E11 is in the heme pocket, providing an additional block to oxygen binding. Movement of the porphyrin ring relative to the heme-linked histidine results in a narrowing of the pocket between helices F and H into which the phenolic group of tyrosine HC2 fits, which leads to its ejection. Rotation of this group distorts the carboxyl-terminal amino acids so that the salt bridges are no longer possible, and they rupture.

Each subunit undergoes change in the tertiary structure with successive oxygenation, as described above; after two or three of them have done so, there is a change in the quaternary structure. This change involves a rotation of the two halves of the molecules ($\alpha\beta$ subunits) relative to one another, and a "sliding" occurs at the $\alpha_1\beta_2$ and $\alpha_2\beta_1$ interfaces (Fig. 3.5).

The equilibrium between the R and T conformations can be influenced by a number of small molecules that bind at specific sites. These *heterotropic* or *allosteric* effectors are mainly hydrogen ion (H^+), chloride (Cl^-), 2,3-DPG (within the red cell), and carbon dioxide (CO_2), but many other compounds bind to hemoglobin as well.

3.2 The Oxygen Equilibrium Curve

The relationship between the fractional saturation of hemoglobin with oxygen and the oxygen physically dissolved in solution (oxygen partial pressure, PO_2) under equilibrium conditions is the familiar oxygen equilibrium curve (OEC) of hemoglobin (Fig. 3.8). Its position is often represented by the value P_{50}, the oxygen partial pressure at half-saturation. If oxygen affinity increases, the OEC shifts left (reduced P_{50}). If oxygen affinity decreases, the OEC shifts right (increased P_{50}).

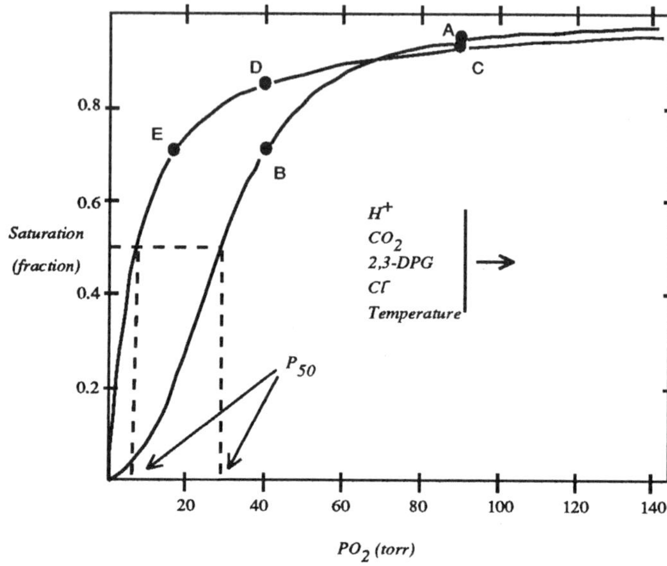

Figure 3.8. The normal blood and myoglobin oxygen equilibrium curves. P_{50} is the PO_2 at which hemoglobin is half-saturated with O_2. The principal effectors that alter the position and shape of the curve are indicated. Note that although both the hemoglobin and myoglobin curves allow saturation of about 95% at normal alveolar oxygen (*A,C*), hemoglobin unloads 23% of its O_2 (*B*) and myoglobin, only 7% (*D*) at 40 torr. In order for myoglobin to deliver 23% of bound O_2, a venous PO_2 of about 16 torr would result in this example (point E).

The principal physiologic effectors of hemoglobin function within the red cell, the molecules that cause such shifts, are H^+, 2,3-DPG, and CO_2. Other effectors, Cl^- and adenosine triphosphate (ATP), also decrease oxygen affinity, but their physiologic roles are minor. The OEC is very sensitive to temperature. The effect of H^+ is called the *Bohr effect*, and is illustrated in Figure 3.9. This figure shows that the position of the OEC is affected by pH. Note that the effect on unmodified hemoglobin is stronger than on the chemically modified hemoglobin. This will be discussed in more detail in a subsequent chapter, but it illustrates that when the molecule is modified chemically, the T to R transition is altered; this alteration is manifest in a reduced Bohr effect.

The sigmoid shape of the hemoglobin OEC is of great importance because it allows the normal loading and unloading of oxygen under

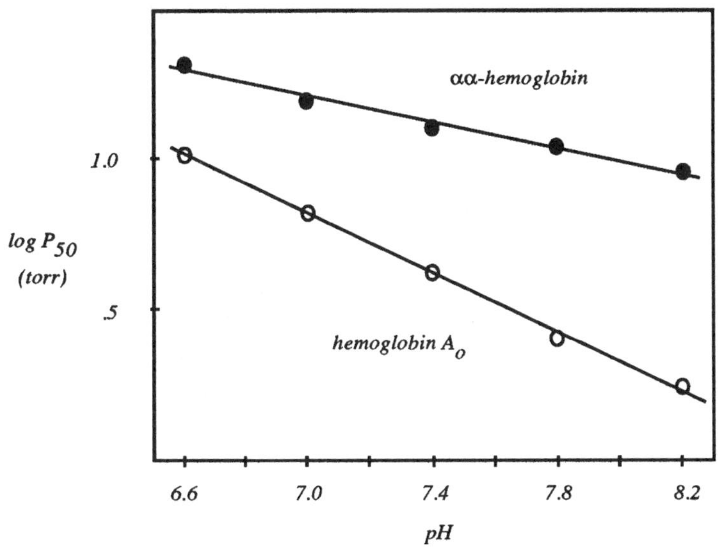

Figure 3.9. The Bohr effect. Hemoglobin modified by cross-linking the α chains has about half the pH dependence of P_{50} (slope = -0.22) of unmodified human hemoglobin A_o (slope = -0.50). *Source:* Vandegriff et al. (1989).

physiologic conditions (Hill 1910). Myoglobin, isolated α and β chains of hemoglobin, and αβ subunits bind oxygen with such high affinity that no effective release of oxygen could occur in tissue. This is illustrated in Figure 3.8, which compares the equilibrium curves for hemoglobin and myoglobin under identical conditions. The oxygen tension in the human alveolus is about 90 torr and in resting tissues, about 40 torr. It is apparent from the figure that at 40 torr hemoglobin can release about 23 percent of its oxygen load. If myoglobin were the respiratory pigment in blood, the oxygen tension in the tissues would have to reach about 16 torr before an equivalent amount of oxygen could be released. Since the oxygen affinity of α or β hemoglobin chains (or of αβ) is approximately that of myoglobin, we can see that the tetrameric structure of hemoglobin is necessary for its suitably low oxygen affinity.

Although hemoglobin also acts as a buffer inside the red cell, the reciprocal transport of the respiratory gases, O_2 and CO_2, between tissues and lungs is its main function. The molecular properties underlying these functions are the cooperative binding of oxygen to heme sites, the Bohr effect, and the interactions of small molecules that alter oxygen binding. All these properties are closely interrelated with extraordinary intricacy.

3.3 Equilibrium Models

3.3.1 Empirical Description: Hill Model

Early physiologists observed the sigmoid nature of the OEC and concluded that oxygen binding increased during progressive oxygenation (Fig. 3.8). They felt that this reflected interaction among heme sites so that oxygen binding to one made binding at the next more likely. They called this phenomenon *cooperativity*. Hill's empirical equation (Hill 1910) is

$$log(Y\ /\ (1-Y)) \ = n\ log(p) + k \tag{1}$$

which relates hemoglobin saturation (Y) to oxygen tension (p). The constant k is the y axis intercept. When plotted according to this equation, the major portion of the OEC falls on a straight line with slope (n) proportional to the degree of cooperativity. It was found that n for hemoglobin was about 3 and for myoglobin, devoid of cooperativity, 1. This mathematical model provides no information about the mechanism of oxygen binding, but the use of Hill's parameter, n, as an index of cooperativity has persisted in the literature.

3.3.2 Partially Liganded Intermediates: Adair Model

A more general approach to the quantitation of the oxygenation of hemoglobin was made by Gilbert Adair, who recognized that hemoglobin is made up of four subunits, each of which could bind a single oxygen molecule (Adair 1925a). He derived equations for the stepwise oxygenation of hemoglobin:

$$Hb(O_2)_i + O_2 \leftrightarrow Hb(O_2)_{i+1} \tag{2}$$

where i ranges from 0 to 3, and the association equilibrium constants for the reactions could be represented as

$$K_i = \frac{[Hb(O_2)_{i+1}]}{[Hb(O_2)_i][O_2]} \tag{3}$$

Combining the four resulting equations,

$$Y = \frac{K_1\,p + K_1K_2\,p^2 + K_1K_2K_3\,p^3 + K_1K_2K_3K_4\,p^4}{1+4(K_1\,p + K_1K_2\,p^2 + K_1K_2K_3\,p^3 + K_1K_2K_3K_4\,p^4)} \tag{4}$$

where Y is fractional saturation of hemoglobin with oxygen, K is the equilibrium constant for the individual combination of oxygen with hemoglobin, and p is the partial pressure of oxygen. Equation 4 is usually simplified by combining the equilibrium constants:

$$Y = \frac{a_1\,p + a_2\,p^2 + a_3\,p^3 + a_4\,p^4}{1+4(1+a_1\,p + a_2\,p^2 + a_3\,p^3 + a_4\,p^4)} \tag{5}$$

The new parameters (a) are called *Adair parameters.*

One difficulty with the Adair scheme is that it is too general: unique values of a are difficult to determine experimentally, and therefore the K values are nearly impossible because of the high degree of interdependence among the parameters (Roughton et al. 1972; Winslow et al. 1977). In addition, the model is structure independent and thus is of little help in conceptualizing structure-function relationships. Nevertheless, it is possible to describe the OEC by the Adair parameters, and this has practical utility even if the values are not unique (Winslow et al. 1983).

Using experimentally derived values for the Adair parameters of human blood (Winslow et al. 1983), the concentration of each of the partially liganded intermediates can be calculated. As shown in Figure 3.10, the concentration of $Hb(O_2)_3$ is very low at all saturation levels. This is consistent with the notion that molecules undergo a conformational switch when the third oxygen binds such that binding of the fourth oxygen is almost instantaneous.

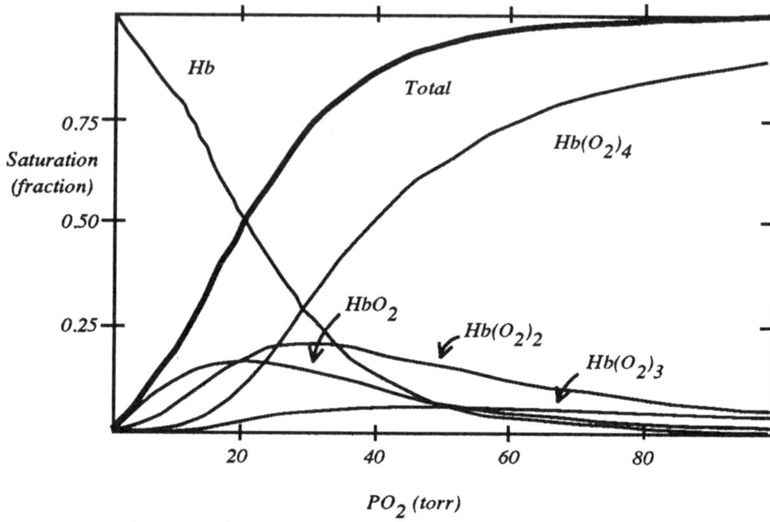

Figure 3.10. Partially liganded O_2 intermediates calculated from the Adair parameters for the stepwise oxygenation of hemoglobin. Note that the triply liganded species ($Hb(O_2)_3$) is predicted to be present in very small amounts.

Unless the affinities of the α and β chain oxygen-binding sites are identical, the scheme proposed by Adair is an oversimplification since a variety of intermediate molecules is possible (Fig. 3.11). Low-temperature quenching techniques have been developed by Michele Perrella and co-workers (Perrella and Rossi-Bernardi 1981) which verify the presence and amounts of partially liganded intermediates. The intermediates shown in Figure 3.10 are, in fact, present, and their concentrations are in general agreement with the predictions from the Adair model (Perrella 1988).

3.3.3 Allosteric Effectors: Two-state Model

Since the elucidation of the exact structure of hemoglobin, several mechanistic theories for the influence of the allosteric effectors (H^+, 2,3-DPG, CO_2, Cl^-, for example) have been proposed (Antonini and Brunori 1971), but the work of Monod, Wyman, and Changeaux (1965), supported by the structural work of Perutz (Bolton and Perutz 1970), is the

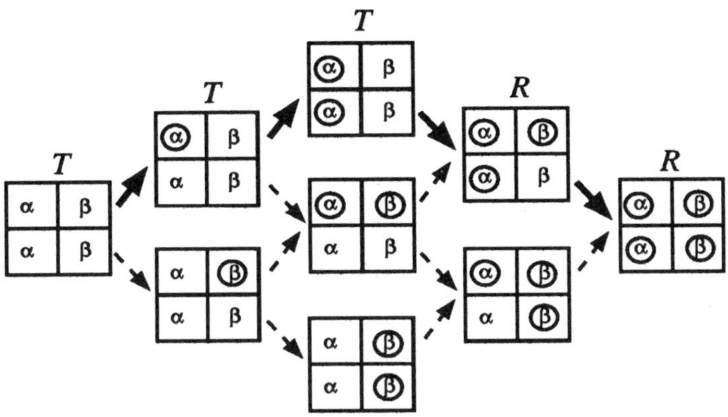

Figure 3.11. The possible structural varieties of partially liganded oxygenation intermediates, assuming that α and β heme sites have unique binding affinities. The α_2 - cooperon model suggests the preferred path shown with *solid arrows*. In this case, the T to R transition would occur as the third O_2 is bound, and the fourth binds almost instantaneously.

basis of the most widely applicable model.

According to the two-state model, each of the two hemoglobin conformations (*R* and *T*) has a unique oxygen affinity. The association equilibrium constants for their reactions with oxygen are K_R and K_T. The ratio of these constants,

$$C = K_T / K_R \tag{6}$$

is about 0.01 for human hemoglobin A; that is, the affinity of molecules in the R conformation is much greater than for those in the T conformation. The constant C is characteristic of a given hemoglobin structure. The essence of the allosteric theory is that the equilibrium between the two conformations in the deoxy state

$$Hb_R \leftrightarrow Hb_T \tag{7}$$

given by the allosteric constant

$$L = [Hb]^T / [Hb]^R \tag{8}$$

is influenced by a number of allosteric effectors. These small molecules react with hemoglobin at nonheme sites in such a way as to stabilize the T conformation. Thus, the overall reactivity of a mixture of R and T hemoglobin molecules toward oxygen will depend on the position of the R–T equilibrium. Monod, Wyman, and Changeaux (1965) related the allosteric constant L to oxygen tension (p) and fractional saturation of hemoglobin with oxygen (Y):

$$Y = \frac{LK_T p(1+K_T p)^3 + K_R p(1+K_R p)^3}{L(1+K_T p)^4 + (1+K_R p)^4} \tag{9}$$

Of fundamental importance in this model is that the T state is physically constrained to a much greater degree than the R state. With successive oxygenation of the heme groups the stability of the T structure decreases, and as a result the molecules undergo a transition to the R state with the release of the constraints and an increase in oxygen affinity. For deoxyhemoglobin the equilibrium is almost entirely on the T side. It is the shift from T to R during oxygenation which accounts for cooperativity. For normal hemoglobin, most of the molecules probably shift from T to R between binding of the second and third oxygen molecules; hence the OEC is steepest in its middle portion.

Although the two-state model may not apply in all circumstances it has been very useful in explaining certain properties of some abnormal hemoglobins. Many of them can be viewed as structural alterations that affect the value of L by favoring either the T (low affinity) or R (high affinity) conformation.

3.3.4 Subunit Heterogeneity: The Cooperon Model

Experiments using concentrated hemoglobin (Gill et al. 1987; Robert, Fall, and Gill 1988) and whole blood (Winslow et al. 1977) showed that when the data were analyzed according to the Adair scheme, the parameter a_3 (Equation 5) became unmeasurable and approached zero or even negative values. This prompted the formulation of a third model that is really a special case of the two-state model (Brunori, Coletta, and DiCera 1986; DiCera, Robert, and Gill 1987). This model proposes that in the T state tetramer oxygen binds preferentially to the α chain. Interaction between α chains may lead to cooperativity within the T state but when the quaternary transition to the R state occurs, the affinities of both α and β chains for oxygen are equal and act as a unit (cooperon).

The cooperon model introduces a new parameter, γ, that defines the chain interactions in the T state. When γ is greater than 1, interaction is positive; it is negative when γ is less than 1. When γ = 1, α chains are independent of each other. Mathematically, the α_2 cooperon model can be written

$$Y = \frac{L(K_T p + \gamma\ K_T^2 p^2) + 2K_R p(1 + K_R p)^3}{L(1 + 2K_T p + \gamma\ K_T^2 p^2) + 2(1 + K_R p)^4} \qquad (10)$$

Note that this expression has four parameters, like the Adair equation.

The cooperon model suggests an explanation for the low population of triply ligated intermediates of oxygenation (i.e., zero value of a_3): binding of the first two oxygen molecules would be to the two α chains (α_2 cooperon) because the affinity of the β sites is negligible in the T state. For the third oxygen to bind, the molecule must switch to the R state, in which the affinity of both β sites is high, and the population of molecules with only one β site saturated is very low (Fig. 3.11).

3.3.5 The Bohr Effect

Bohr observed that the position of the blood OEC along the abscissa was affected by changes in CO_2 partial pressure (Bohr, Hasselbalch, and Krogh 1904); that is, when the pH was lowered (or PCO_2 raised), the oxygen affinity of the blood decreased (increased P_{50}). The separate effects of H^+ and CO_2 have now been elucidated (Kilmartin and Rossi-Bernardi 1973). They are similar qualitatively, but the effect of H^+ (now properly called the pH effect) is much stronger than the CO_2 effect in lowering oxygen affinity.

According to the two-state model of hemoglobin function, H^+ shifts the R–T equilibrium toward T, stabilizing that structure. The stereochemical interpretation of this phenomenon is H^+ participation in opening and closing the salt bridges involving the carboxyl-terminal residues.

The pK values of the imidazoles of histidine HC3(146)β and of valine Nal(1)α are lowered in oxyhemoglobin as a result of the rupture of the salt bridges in which they participate. This change in pK leads to a release of protons during the transition from T to R. Experiments with mutant and chemically modified hemoglobins suggest that these groups account for about two-thirds of the alkaline Bohr effect (Kilmartin, Fogg, and Rossi-Bernardi 1975).

3.3.6 2,3-Diphosphoglycerate

The normal intracellular constituent 2,3-DPG (and, to a lesser extent, ATP) is very important in the regulation of the blood OEC (Benesch and Benesch 1967). 2,3-DPG, a metabolic intermediate in the glycolytic pathway, is a normal constituent of human red blood cells. Under conditions of diminished oxygen availability (such as anemia or hypoxia), its concentration increases, shifting the blood OEC to the right. If arterial oxygenation is normal, this facilitates transfer of oxygen to the tissues. The regulatory mechanisms that govern the concentration of 2,3-DPG are not completely understood, but alkalosis in response to hyperventilation is probably an important factor (Lenfant and Sullivan 1971).

2,3-DPG can bind to deoxyhemoglobin in a molar ratio of 1:1 and by doing so, further constrain the T conformation, leading to an additional shift of the R–T equilibrium toward T, lowering the oxygen affinity. Salt bridges involving the free amino groups of valine NA1(1)β and the imidazoles of histidine H21(143)β are probably the most important binding sites (Arnone 1972). In deoxyhemoglobin, 2,3-DPG lies in the central cavity of the molecule and is coordinated to the groups mentioned above plus the ε-amino groups of lysine EF6(82)β. On transition to the R structure, the valines move apart, the H helices move together, and 2,3-DPG drops out. As in the effects of the other salt bridges in the deoxy structure, 2,3-DPG increases the alkaline Bohr effect.

3.3.7 Carbon Dioxide Binding

Finally, CO_2 can bind to the α-amino groups of the amino-terminal amino acids with a resultant decrease of oxygen affinity (Kilmartin and Rossi-Bernardi 1973). This binding is diminished in the presence of 2,3-DPG since both 2,3-DPG and CO_2 can bind to the β-chain amino-terminal amino group. Such competition does not occur for the α-chain amino terminus since 2,3-DPG does not bind there.

3.4 Symmetry

Graphically (Fig. 3.12), a symmetric OEC is one in which the area above the curve from its central point to infinite oxygen tension is equal

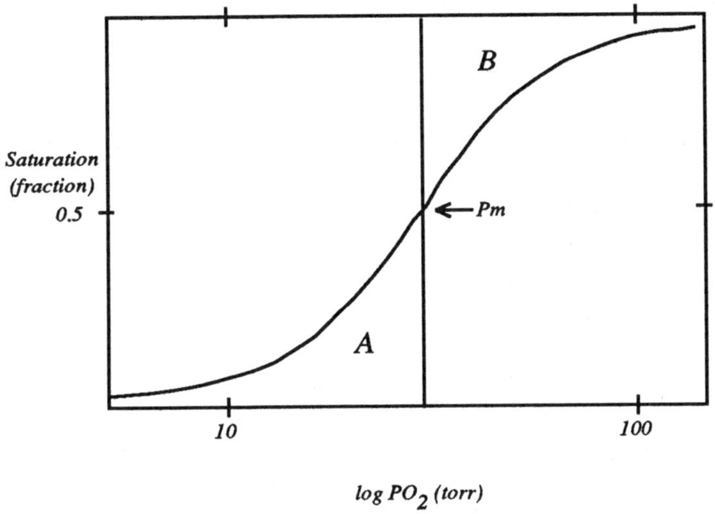

Figure 3.12. **Symmetry of oxygen binding. The median ligand concentration (*Pm*) is defined graphically as the PO_2 at which a *vertical line* passes through the curve such that area *A* is equal to area *B*. Reduced cooperativity would be manifest by clockwise rotation of the curve about *Pm*.**

to the area below the curve from 0 to its central point (Wyman 1964). The oxygen tension at which these two areas are equal is the median ligand pressure, Pm, and for a symmetric curve, P_{50} = Pm. To quantitate this concept, Allen, Guthe, and Wyman (1950) defined symmetry as the condition $K_1K_4 = K_2K_3$. Roughton and co-workers (1972) showed that for a symmetric OEC, the *Wyman factor,* W, should approximate 1:

$$W = (a_1 / a_3)^2 a_4 \tag{11}$$

Weber (1982) investigated symmetry for hemoglobin solutions and defined a descriptive parameter:

$$A = ln(K_1K_4 / K_2K_3) \tag{12}$$

This parameter has a positive value when $K_1K_4 > K_2K_3$ and a negative value when $K_1K_4 < K_2K_3$. Weber proposed that positive values of A are associated with efficient unloading of oxygen from hemoglobin, whereas negative values are better for scavenging oxygen in the lung. He calculated positive values of A ranging from 0.44 for purified hemoglobin to 4.59 for hemoglobin with maximally reduced oxygen affinity.

In contrast, using the best whole blood data available to him, Roughton concluded that W for whole blood is about 85, a value that did not seem to be consistent with any known model of hemoglobin function. More recent data (Winslow, Winslow, and Samaja 1991) allow a calculation of W for whole blood which is about 9. Given the errors in the determination of the parameters, this is probably not significantly different from 1 and is consistent with the notion that within the red cell very little triply liganded hemoglobin is present, probably because it is almost completely in the high affinity (R) conformation. Calculation of Weber's parameter for whole blood gives a value of 2.16 (Winslow, Winslow, and Samaja 1991). This positive value is consistent with Weber's hypothesis that the human blood system is geared to efficient oxygen release in tissues. Experimental confirmation will await systematic studies of the effect of manipulation of the OEC on tissue oxygenation.

3.5 Oxidation of Hemoglobin

It is usually thought that lowering the oxygen pressure accelerates oxidation of heme iron, because of reduced stability of the T structure. Levy and co-workers have studied the rates of autooxidation of hemoglobin at various oxygen tensions and found that fully oxygenated hemoglobin is especially resistant to oxidation. The partially liganded T state hemoglobin with one ligand oxidizes faster, but the major source of oxidation is the triply liganded R state (Zhang, Rifkind, and Levy 1990). This would explain why when the OEC shifts right, oxidation seems faster.

Chapter 4

Oxygen Transport by Hemoglobin

In simple single-cell animals, the transport of oxygen from air to mitochondria is a diffusive process, and no circulation is needed. As organisms increase in size and complexity, however, the distances for diffusion are too great, and a circulation is required. Invertebrates transport oxygen in a circulating hemolymph that contains either hemocyanin (van Holde and van Bruggen 1971), a copper-containing protein, or hemerythrin (Klotz 1971), an iron-containing protein. In both of these, the metal atom is coordinated directly to the protein. In higher organisms such as man, the transport of oxygen is far more complex, with hemoglobin packaged in cells that are transported in the blood by alternate exposure to air in the lung and to capillary beds in tissues.

Red blood cells are uniquely suited to the task of oxygen transport for several important reasons. First, they contain a high concentration (about 35 g/dl) of hemoglobin, capable of carrying about 47 volumes of oxygen per 100 volumes of hemoglobin. Hemoglobin at this concentration could not circulate, so it is packaged in cells that themselves occupy about 45 percent of the volume of blood. Thus, the overall oxygen capacity is about 18 volumes per 100 volumes of blood; blood without red cells would contain only about 2 volumes per 100 volumes. Second, red blood cells are deformable; they can squeeze into capillaries that are smaller in width than the dimension of the cells themselves. This ensures a minimal distance for diffusion of oxygen from the alveolar space of the lung to hemoglobin or from hemoglobin to sites of tissue respiration. Third, as discussed in the preceding chapter, hemoglobin binds oxygen cooperatively. This means that very small changes in oxygen tension result in large amounts of oxygen either taken up in the lung or released in the tissues. Finally, hemoglobin demonstrates a Bohr effect: local conditions of pH and carbon dioxide affect the oxygen-binding behavior of hemoglobin in ways that are favorable for oxygen transport.

Since the supply of oxygen is critical to organ function and therefore survival, it is expected that the physiologic mechanisms that ensure this supply are complex and redundant. This chapter will consider the quantitative interaction of some of these red cell properties with other physiologic determinants of oxygen transport. These concepts will form a foundation upon which to consider the pertinent physiologic requirements for a blood substitute. We will examine the oxygen transport system perturbed by hypoxia. This is extremely useful because the delivery of oxygen to tissues is the essence of blood substitute development, and the study of the reaction of the body to hypoxia will demonstrate the needed properties of these solutions.

4.1 Determinants of Oxygen Transport

4.1.1 Fick Equation

Overall oxygen transport is given by the Fick equation:

$$\dot{V}O_2 = C(a-\bar{v})O_2 \times \dot{Q} \tag{1}$$

where $\dot{V}O_2$ is the rate of oxygen uptake, $(a\text{-}\bar{v})O_2$ is the difference between the arterial and venous oxygen contents, and $\dot{Q}$ is the cardiac output. Arterial oxygen content is determined by the hemoglobin concentration of the blood, the ability of the lung to transfer oxygen from alveolar air to blood, and the ability of the blood to take up oxygen from the alveolar membrane. Cardiac output is determined to a large extent by the level of oxygen demand (work load) and by the resistance to flow in the arterial circulation, which is influenced in turn by the bulk viscosity of the blood.

These relationships are extraordinarily complex (Fig. 4.1): consider, for example, that the uptake of oxygen in the lung is influenced by the oxygen affinity of the red cells. The oxygen affinity, or P_{50}, as discussed in Chapter 3, is a function not only of the intrinsic oxygen affinity of hemoglobin but also of pH, 2,3-diphosphoglycerate (2,3-DPG) content of the red cells, and carbon dioxide tension. The pH is itself determined by the hemoglobin concentration (hemoglobin is a buffer of hydrogen ions) and carbon dioxide tension.

The transfer of oxygen from the red cell to tissue mitochondria must pass through several phases, shown in Figure 4.2. After release from hemoglobin, oxygen must diffuse to the red cell membrane and pass

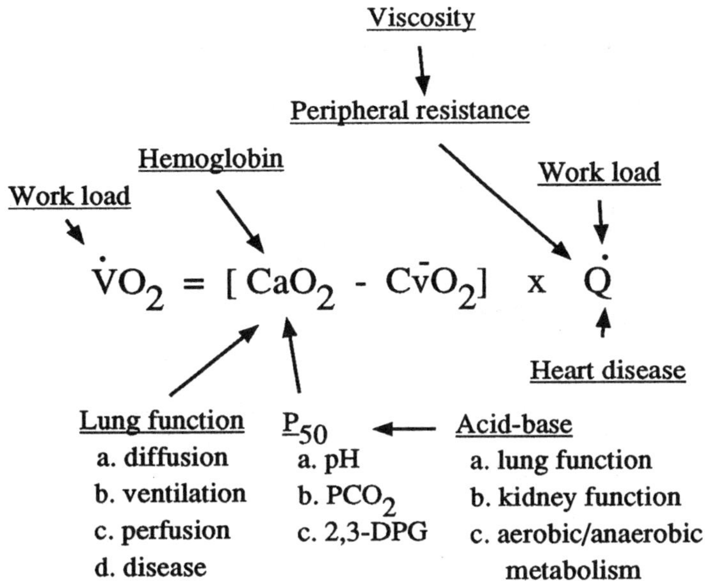

Figure 4.1. Interactions of the determinants of oxygen transport.

through it. The plasma contains very little oxygen compared to red cells, because of the low solubility. Immediately surrounding the red cell is a layer of unstirred plasma which moves with the red cell and which represents a stagnant layer. Diffusion through this area is slow. Oxygen must then diffuse through the stirred (moving) plasma phase, to the endothelial membrane, through it, into tissue, and then through tissue to the mitochondrion.

It is almost impossible to consider all the diverse ways in which these variables can simultaneously interact in the body to determine overall oxygen transport. The various barriers to diffusion shown in Figure 4.2 are very difficult to quantitate, but some generalizations can be made regarding the overall transport of oxygen in blood. Mathematical models are extremely useful to aid in appreciating the integration of the overall system.

4.1.2 Oxygen Affinity

It is clear that the oxygen-binding behavior of hemoglobin can affect

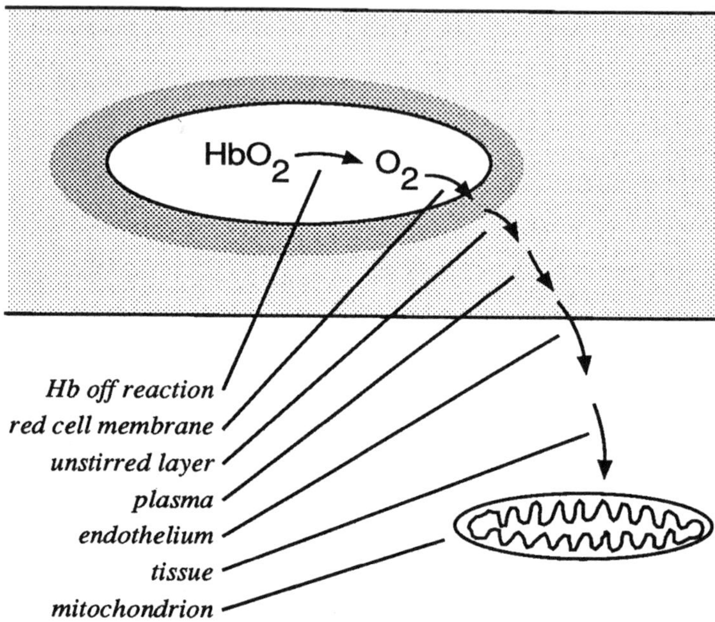

Figure 4.2. The various barriers to diffusion of oxygen as it transfers from the red blood cell to the mitochondrion.

overall oxygen transport because certain genetic alterations in the molecule may lead to polycythemia (Winslow and Anderson 1982). Furthermore, an extreme left shift in the oxygen equilibrium curve caused by severe respiratory alkalosis was an essential feature in oxygen transport on the summit of Mount Everest (Winslow, Samaja, and West 1984). The effect of reduced affinity has been shown by a number of authors to improve oxygen delivery to tissues when arterial oxygenation is adequate (Woodson, Wranne and Detter 1973).

Experimental demonstration that changes in the position or shape of the oxygen equilibrium curve may affect oxygen transport has been difficult, and therefore theoretical studies of the problem have been based on simplified models of hemoglobin oxygenation (Neville 1976; Bencowitz, Wagner, and West 1982; Willford, Hill, and Moores 1982). Other known red cell properties that affect oxygen transport include the rates of binding of physiologic ligands (O_2, CO_2, H^+, 2,3-DPG), buffering capacity, the barrier to diffusion presented by the red cell membrane, the layer of unstirred plasma immediately surrounding it, and the hematocrit-dependent blood viscosity (Winslow 1985).

The traditional view is that shifting the oxygen equilibrium curve to the right (higher P_{50}) facilitates oxygen unloading in tissue sites. However, in certain situations the opposite could be true. For example, Joseph Barcroft et al. (1923) believed that increased oxygen affinity (left-shifted oxygen equilibrium curve) was important in adaptation to high altitude. Their reasoning was based on analogy with the placental circulation, in which fetal blood has a higher affinity than that of the mother. The modification of hemoglobin to increase its affinity conveys superior survival on hypoxic rats (Eaton, Skelton, and Berger 1974), and mutant hemoglobins with increased affinity may precondition subjects to hypoxia (Hebbel et al. 1978). On the summit of Mount Everest, the P_{50} of whole blood is about 19 torr, protecting arterial saturation (Winslow, Samaja, and West 1984).

An increase in 2,3-DPG is usually thought to augment oxygen delivery by a right shift of the oxygen equilibrium curve, but this is probably only true in normoxia (sea level). At higher altitudes, because of the diffusion limitation to oxygen uptake in the lung, decreased oxygen affinity seems to limit uptake. Whether or not this is offset by tissue unloading remains to be seen because too few data are available to indicate how low venous oxygen tension can drop under hypoxic conditions. At this point it seems that the 2,3-DPG effect is a sea level mechanism, not suited to oxygen delivery in hypoxia.

The rate of oxygen uptake by red cells is important in the lung, but it is difficult to measure. The importance of the layer of unstirred plasma surrounding the red cell membrane in vivo is still not appreciated (Vandegriff and Olson 1984). It appears, however, that the reaction of oxygen with hemoglobin itself is not rate limiting.

4.1.3 A Model for Red Blood Cell Oxygen Uptake

A mathematical model that is able to present graphically the interaction of the various factors that determine the uptake of oxygen by red cells illustrates these concepts (Winslow 1985). Although it may be more useful to compute gas exchange along tissue capillaries, this is a more complex procedure because of the additional countercurrent exchange that occurs between arterioles and venules. In our model, we first estimated the mixed venous acid-base conditions, the cardiac output, and the oxygen equilibrium curves under arterial and venous conditions. Then over discrete finite time elements, new conditions were estimated as the red cell traversed the pulmonary capillary. Oxygen tensions could then be calculated as the red cell progressed through the pulmonary capillary (Fig. 4.3).

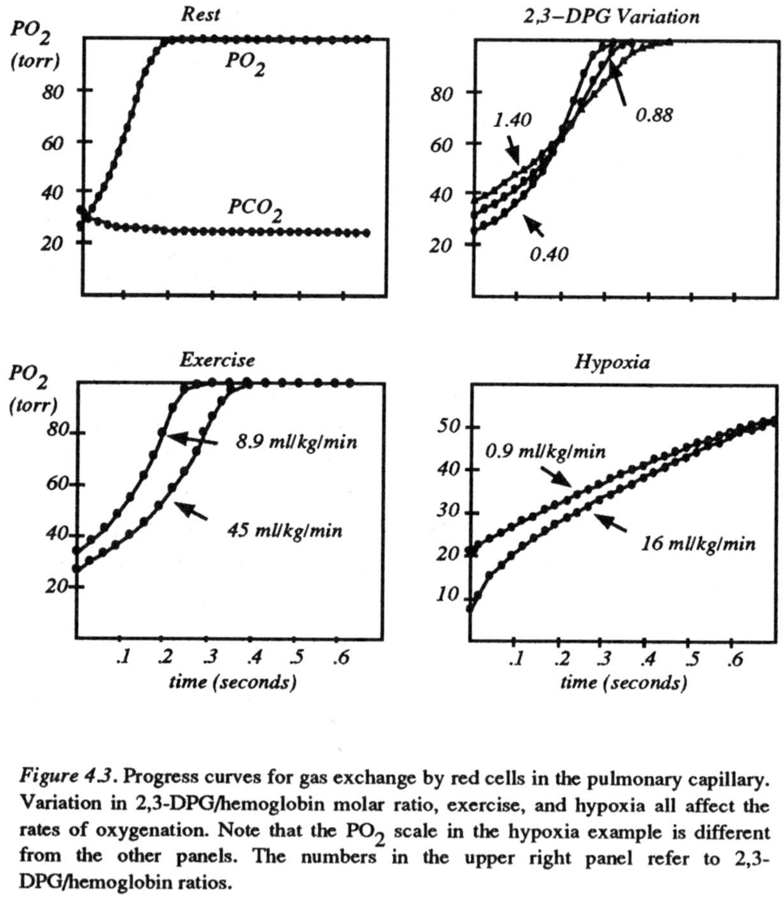

Figure 4.3. Progress curves for gas exchange by red cells in the pulmonary capillary. Variation in 2,3-DPG/hemoglobin molar ratio, exercise, and hypoxia all affect the rates of oxygenation. Note that the PO_2 scale in the hypoxia example is different from the other panels. The numbers in the upper right panel refer to 2,3-DPG/hemoglobin ratios.

Our procedure differs from previous ones because we are not restricted by the Hill equation to describe the oxygen equilibrium curve, which is accurate only over a narrow saturation range. We also consider the cardiac output dependence on hematocrit and oxygen uptake. A new oxygen equilibrium curve is calculated at each step so that the new saturation can be used in the acid-base calculation.

Oxygen uptake progress curves were computed at hematocrits from 5 to 85 percent over the 2,3-DPG/hemoglobin ratio range 0.3–1.5 mol/mol. At each 2,3-DPG/hemoglobin, curves were calculated at each hematocrit in steps of 5 percent. The constraints used were: (1) that venous oxygen content and partial pressure must be positive; (2) that end capillary oxygen tension must reach the measured arterial oxygen tension; and (3) that acid-base conditions must be found such that arterial and venous base excess were the same. When condition 2 was not satisfied, oxygen uptake was decreased by 10 percent of its initial value, and the computations were retried. If all conditions could not be met, a value of 0 was assigned to mixed venous oxygen tension, and the process continued.

To study the interaction of red cell oxygen affinity with hematocrit and viscosity (cardiac output), triaxial (hematocrit, 2,3-DPG/hemoglobin, $P\bar{v}O_2$) plots were made. This model was validated with data collected in humans with various hematocrits performing different levels of work at elevated altitudes (Winslow 1985).

4.1.4 2,3-Diphosphoglycerate/hemoglobin Molar Ratio

The study of variations in the 2,3-DPG/hemoglobin molar ratio is a much more instructive procedure than simply shifting the oxygen equilibrium curve without altering its shape (Bencowitz, Wagner, and West 1982) because under physiologic conditions 2,3-DPG/hemoglobin is the main modulator of the position and shape of the oxygen equilibrium curve (see Fig. 3.7). Increasing 2,3-DPG/hemoglobin has the effect of increasing mixed venous oxygen tension and also of increasing the time required for oxygenation, since the oxygen affinity is decreased. During exercise these two effects are illustrated more clearly. As 2,3-DPG/hemoglobin increases, the time to oxygenate approaches the pulmonary capillary transit time, and at a 2,3-DPG/hemoglobin ratio of 1.4 mol per mol of hemoglobin, the model cannot satisfy the input conditions without decreasing the rate of oxygen uptake.

In hypoxia, the effect of 2,3-DPG/hemoglobin is even more apparent (Fig. 4.3). At rest, decreasing 2,3-DPG/hemoglobin allows the blood to become oxygenated within the allowed transit time, but increasing even above 0.4 mol/mol leads to arterial desaturation. This can become limiting in exercise; mixed venous oxygen tension must decrease to dangerously low levels at all 2,3-DPG/hemoglobin ratios, but when 2,3-DPG/hemoglobin is less than 0.4 mol/mol, arterial desaturation occurs.

4.1.5 Hematocrit

With increasing hematocrit (and viscosity), cardiac output decreases, producing lower mixed venous oxygen tension. However, the time allowed for capillary transit increases, which could be of some benefit to overall gas transport.

4.1.6 Exercise

Exercise increases the oxygen requirement and therefore the cardiac output. Increased cardiac output decreases the pulmonary "dwell" time and therefore the time allowed for oxygen uptake by red cells. Ordinarily this is not a problem, but in extremely high cardiac output states, the time allowed in the lung may not be sufficient to oxygenate red cells, resulting in arterial desaturation.

4.1.7 Hypoxia

The main effect of hypoxia is to decrease the oxygen gradient between pulmonary alveolus and capillary blood. Thus the rate of transfer will decrease. Again, at rest, this is not a serious problem, but in exercise or other states of increased oxygen demand, oxygenation could be severely limited.

4.1.8 Multiple Effects

To consider these effects individually is instructive but not realistic. In fact, they vary together, and this can be visualized by the exercise of optimizing the mixed venous oxygen tension. To do this, we calculate oxygen uptake for various conditions and then the arterial and mixed venous oxygen tension that would be needed to satisfy the required rate. This is useful to the extent that mixed venous oxygen tension is a useful indicator of tissue oxygenation.

Figure 4.4 shows triaxial surfaces that relate hematocrit and 2,3-DPG (hence P_{50}) to mixed venous oxygen tension under different conditions of oxygen transfer. As the figure shows, mixed venous oxygen tension drops at high and low hematocrit, and increasing 2,3-DPG (elevated P_{50}) helps to a small degree. During exercise 2,3-DPG still has some effect, but the effect of increased hematocrit is a little sharper. In hypoxia it seems that increasing 2,3-DPG has a negative effect since its increase actually decreases mixed venous oxygen tension. In the combination of hypoxia and exercise the optimal conditions for mixed venous oxygen tension become quite sharp, and severe penalties are paid for deviation from optimal conditions. This analysis makes qualitative sense since it is well known that deviations from normal physiologic responses are poorly tolerated in subjects residing at high altitude (Winslow and Monge 1987).

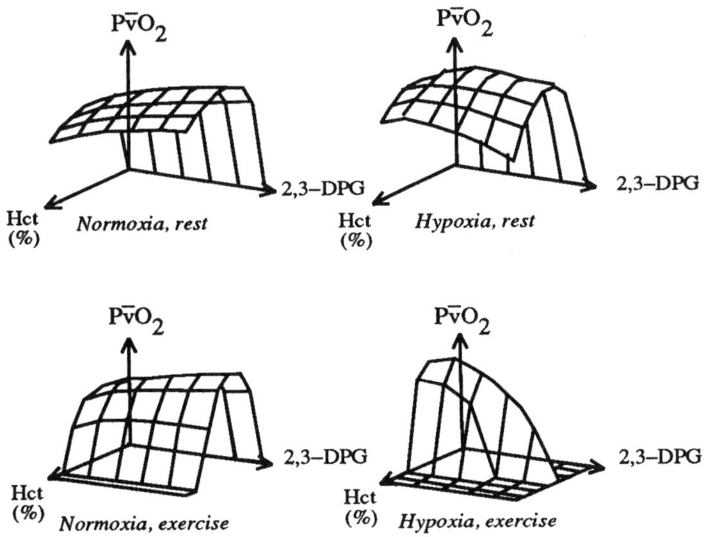

Figure 4.4. Mixed venous PO_2 optimization surfaces for normoxia (rest, exercise) and hypoxia (rest, exercise). Hematocrit range is 5–85 percent, 2,3-DPG/hemoglobin range is 0.3–1.5 mol/mol, and the $P\bar{v}O_2$ range is 0–40 torr. Note that the optima are sharper when the oxygen demand is high or the supply is low.

4.1.9 Rheology

Arthur Guyton and his co-workers (1973) carried out an extensive investigation of the effect of the hematocrit on hemodynamics in the denervated dog and suggested that there is an "optimal hematocrit" for oxygen transport which balances viscosity against oxygen-carrying capacity. In general, an increased hematocrit will increase the vascular resistance to flow, requiring an increased blood pressure and left atrial filling pressure until eventually a new equilibrium among these parameters is reached. Phlebotomy studies in patients with very high hematocrits demonstrate that polycythemia probably contributes to ventilation/perfusion mismatch and arterial desaturation (Winslow et al. 1985).

The relationship between the ability of the blood to transport oxygen, the oxygen-binding properties of hemoglobin, and the flow properties of blood is made somewhat more complex by the fact that whole blood is a non-Newtonian fluid, that is, the apparent viscosity of a suspension of red cells is dependent on the flow rate. In physical terms, the shear stress is dependent on the shear rate. In biologic terms, the vascular resistance to flow is dependent on the rate of blood flow. In contrast, a homogeneous solution such as cell-free hemoglobin is nearly Newtonian; its viscosity does not depend on shear rate.

Introduction of a Newtonian, oxygen-carrying solution to red cell suspensions introduces a new order of complexity. Furthermore, the nature of the hemoglobin modification will be important in determining the qualitative relationships among these curves: polymerized hemoglobin has a higher relative viscosity at an equivalent hemoglobin concentration than unpolymerized hemoglobin. Cerny, Stasiw, and Cerny (1982) used the ratio of hematocrit to viscosity (Chien 1977) to express the "optimal" ratio for mixtures of red cells and hemoglobin. They found a hematocrit of about 22 percent in 6.1 g/dl hemoglobin to be optimal. In contrast, hemoglobin in the absence of red cells does not reach an optimum, but rather the ratio rises indefinitely.

Studies such as those of Cerny need to be extended to the various types of hemoglobin solution currently under study. Such data should be correlated further with in vivo measurements of hemodynamics, along the lines of the work by Guyton and his colleagues, in order to determine the optimal hematologic conditions for hemodilution.

4.1.10 The Balance Between Oxygen Supply and Demand

It is customary to use the shorthand P_{50} to denote characteristics about the ability of a solution to transport oxygen. The above discussion should make it very clear that this is so oversimplified as to be useless. Instead, one would like a parameter that relates the function of a given solution to the ability to maintain metabolism in tissues.

Stainsby and Otis (1964) explored the relationship between the oxygen delivered to tissue and that actually utilized (Fig. 4.5). They found that as oxygen delivery drops, the oxygen uptake is constant until a "critical" point is reached, when uptake falls off precipitously. Probably at this point the cell is faced with the alternatives of lowering its oxygen requirement or drawing upon alternative sources of energy (Gutierrez 1988), and function fails.

Acutely, mammalian tissues have no good method to lower oxygen requirements or to find alternate sources of energy at very high work levels, and so anaerobic metabolism begins, with production of lactic acid. In humans, the actual value of the critical oxygen delivery is about 10 ml/min/kg.

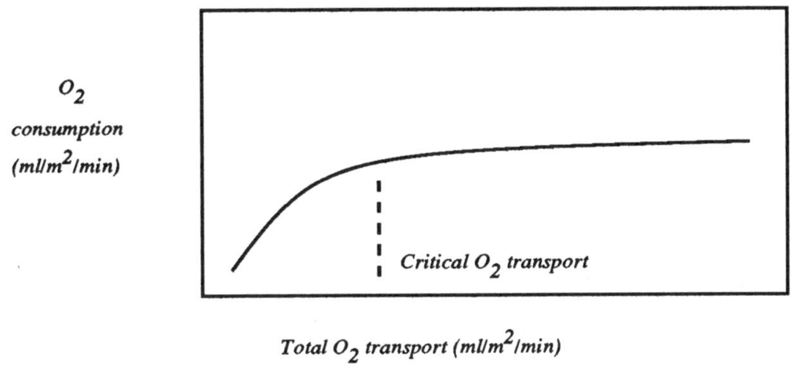

Figure 4.5. Schematic diagram of the relationship between O_2 delivered and O_2 consumption. Oxygen consumption remains constant until the critical oxygen transport is reached, at which point it begins to drop. This plot is a better analysis of the ability of a solution to deliver O_2 than is the oxygen equilibrium curve. *Source*: adapted from Gutierrez (1988).

An interesting study of the critical oxygen delivery was carried out by Cain (1977) who compared decreases in oxygen delivery by either hypoxia or anemia. In both conditions, the oxygen delivery fell to about the same level but in the anemic cases the mixed venous oxygen tension was higher at the critical point. In other words, it was the oxygen *content* (convection), not oxygen *tension* (diffusion), which limited oxygen delivery. This result implies that some kinetic process such as the hemoglobin-oxygen off-reaction might be limiting (Gutierrez 1988).

Analysis of the critical oxygen tension is extremely important because it demonstrates more precisely when dangerous levels of oxygen are reached. Obviously a therapeutic goal of any transfusion of red cells or a hemoglobin-based substitute would be to provide a margin of safety by maintaining oxygen delivery above the critical point.

4.1.11 Blood Substitutes

The oxygen affinity of modified hemoglobin depends on the site and nature of the modification. Figure 4.6 shows examples of solutions with a range of P_{50} values. Hemoglobin-based red cell substitutes may have other beneficial oxygen transport effects that have not been appreciated yet. For example, because of very low viscosity these solutions could perfuse capillary beds that cannot be perfused by red blood cells. In fact, one study of posttrauma patients found that infusion of red cells did not increase oxygen consumption or raise mixed venous oxygen tension in spite of raising the hematocrit (Shah et al. 1982).

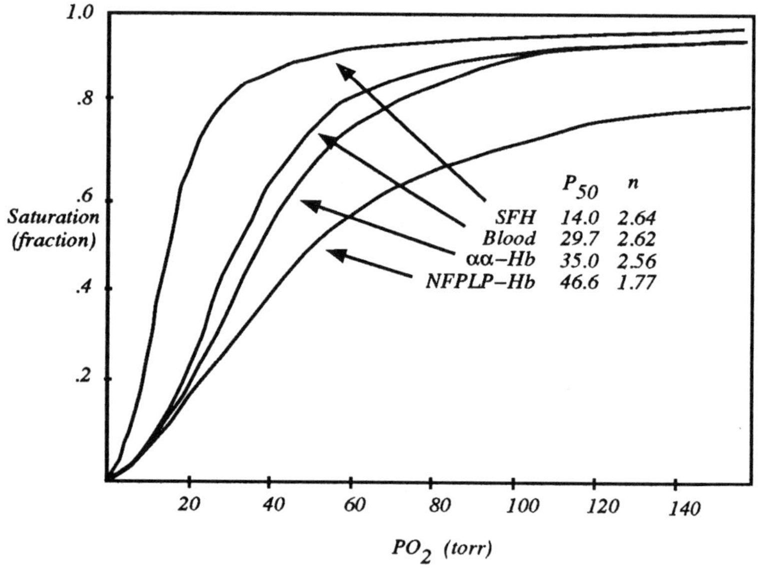

Figure 4.6. Modified hemoglobin solutions with various oxygen affinities. These examples include P_{50} values spanning a range from 14.0 (stroma-free hemoglobin, *SFH*) to 46.6 torr (2-nor-2-formylpyridoxal 5'-phosphate hemoglobin, *NFPLP-Hb*) with different degrees of cooperativity.

Although high-quality products have generally not been available to experimentalists to test various hypotheses about oxygen delivery, particularly in shock or other clinical conditions, some data are available. Thus, Jesch and co-workers (Jesch et al. 1982) studied the oxygen transport properties of hemoglobin and pyridoxylated hemoglobin in resuscitation of posthemorrhagic dogs. They found by direct measurement that the tissue oxygen tension was higher in the animals treated with pyridoxal 5'-phosphate hemoglobin, supporting the claim that reduced oxygen affinity is beneficial to oxygenation of previously ischemic tissue.

Gould and co-workers (Gould et al. 1980) performed total exchange transfusions in eight baboons with either unmodified or pyridoxylated hemoglobin. They found higher mixed venous oxygen tensions in the group that received pyridoxylated hemoglobin compared with the unmodified hemoglobin group when hematocrits fell to below 20 percent. When the hematocrit was 5 percent, the pyridoxylated hemoglobin group had a mixed venous oxygen tension of 31.3 torr whereas in the unmodified hemoglobin group it was 13.8 torr. These data suggest that, as expected, the solution with higher P_{50} allowed a higher tissue oxygen tension than the solution with low P_{50}.

Thus, it seems quite likely that low-viscosity hemoglobin solutions might be able to perfuse tissue better than whole blood. Furthermore, lowered viscosity could lead to raised cardiac output. Free of the red cell, hemoglobin might be able to unload its oxygen in tissues more readily because it would not need to diffuse through the red cell membrane and through the layer of unstirred plasma surrounding it. These beneficial effects could lead to a very efficient transport of oxygen especially in conditions of vascular obstruction or circulatory collapse.

It is too early to know whether other altered properties of hemoglobin, such as CO_2 binding and the Bohr effect, would have physiological implications if the products were used clinically. The binding of CO_2 to αα-Hb is reduced (Vandegriff et al. 1991) as is the Bohr effect of this modified hemoglobin (Vandegriff et al. 1989). It is likely that an altered Bohr effect would have importance only at very high rates of oxygen uptake, however (Wasserman et al. 1991).

Chapter 5
The Modification of Hemoglobin

Joseph Barcroft, as early as 1922, expressed the view that hemoglobin must be packaged inside the red cell because otherwise its viscosity and colloid osmotic pressure would be so high as to cause deranged function (Barcroft 1923). Amberson agreed and extended this view: "We fully agree, however, with Barcroft's argument that the red cell exists to prevent escape of hemoglobin into urine and lymph and to furnish a chemical environment in which hemoglobin may function with maximal efficiency, to which we would add the fact that a major factor in this chemical control is to maintain hemoglobin in its reduced state, electrochemically speaking, so that it is not transformed into physiologically useless methemoglobin" (Amberson 1937, 61).

Hemoglobin has the desirable properties of a high capacity to bind oxygen and to release it cooperatively; this makes it attractive for use as a red cell substitute. However, hemoglobin, free in solution, has several unique properties:

1. Its oxygen affinity is high because outside of the red cell the normal allosteric effector, 2,3-diphosphoglycerate (2,3-DPG), is not present.
2. Its effectiveness as an oxygen carrier is limited because it dissociates into half-molecules ($\alpha\beta$ dimers) that are rapidly removed from the circulation by the kidney after filtration in the glomerulus.
3. Once filtered, a high concentration of protein in the renal tubules can cause tubular obstruction and consequent renal failure.

Thus, to be an effective oxygen carrier in the cell-free state, hemoglobin must be chemically modified to avoid these problems. Some authors have felt that the high colloid osmotic pressure (COP) of cell-free hemoglobin is another problem that needs to be addressed by modification, but as yet there is no agreement as to the optimal COP of a plasma expander (see Chapter 2).

The goals of chemical modification are to decrease the oxygen affinity of hemoglobin and to prevent its dissociation into $\alpha\beta$ dimers. Secondary goals are to perform such modifications with a high yield of product and to obtain derivatives of such purity that specific biologic and chemical properties can be correlated and that toxicologic studies can be carried out and interpreted.

Many studies of the biologic and toxicologic effects of infusions of hemoglobin solutions have been carried out over the past century, many in the hope of developing a hemoglobin-based blood substitute. At this time there is still no product available for clinical use, and an enormous confusing and conflicting literature has accumulated regarding its "toxic" effects. Still, there is no clear demonstration that hemoglobin or its derivatives are toxic. The goal of this chapter is to review some of the current strategies of chemical modification and to try to show some of the reasons why purity of products is both difficult to achieve and of the highest importance. No attempt will be made to present an exhaustive catalogue of all of the chemical modifications of hemoglobin which have been attempted.

5.1 The Reactivity of Hemoglobin

As discussed in detail in Chapter 3, hemoglobin can exist in either of two structural conformations, corresponding to the oxy (R, relaxed) or deoxy (T, tense) states. The key differences between these two structures are that the constrained T state has a much lower oxygen affinity than the R state and that the T state has a lower tendency to dissociate into αβ subunits that can be filtered in the kidneys. Therefore, stabilization by any means of the T conformation would be expected to solve the dual problems of oxygen affinity and renal excretion.

The transition between the T and R states of hemoglobin is also involved deeply in the Bohr effect and cooperativity. Therefore it would be expected that stabilization of either of the two structures would diminish these effects, which have important physiologic consequences. Whether or not this would have *clinical* consequences is not known at present.

Stabilization of the T conformation under normal conditions is illustrated by the reaction of 2,3-DPG (Fig. 5.1). This polyphosphate forms electrostatic, reversible interactions with four amino groups in the 2,3-DPG pocket: 2 α-amino groups of valine NA1(1)β and the two ε-amino groups of lysine EF6(82)α. In the R state the dimensions of the pocket change enough so that 2,3-DPG does not fit as well, and it drops out. Thus, 2,3-DPG preferentially stabilizes the T conformation with the overall effect of reducing oxygen affinity and increasing cooperativity.

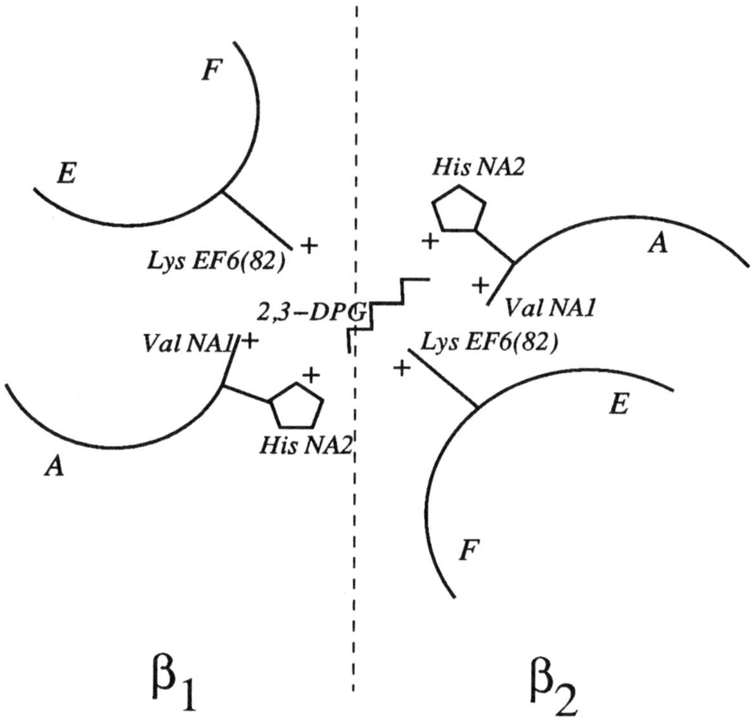

Figure 5.1. Reaction of 2,3-DPG with deoxyhemoglobin. The molecule fits into the central cavity of hemoglobin and forms salt bridges with valine NA(1)β and histidines NA2(2)β and H21(143)β and with lysine EF6(82)β. *Source*: adapted from Arnone (1972).

Analogs of 2,3-DPG can be used to modify hemoglobin by forming permanent, covalent bonds. These are variously effective, depending on their molecular dimensions and their charge. Some of the compounds may react with only one of the reactive amino groups in the 2,3-DPG pocket; others react with all four.

In addition to the 2,3-DPG pocket, human hemoglobin contains forty reactive lysines (ε-amino groups), two α-chain amino-terminal α-amino groups, and two sulfhydryl groups (cysteine F9(93)β). Most of the lysines are on the surface of the molecule, but some are internal, such as lysine G6(99)α. Thus, the groups can be accessed by various cross-linkers and polymerizing agents, especially aldehydes. Although the

Table 5.1. Classes of Hemoglobin Modifications

Class	Examples
Amino-terminal modification	Carbamylation Carboxymethylation Pyridoxylation Acetaldehyde
Lysine EF6(82)β modification	Mono-(3,5-dibromosalicyl)fumarate
Valine NA1(1)β-lysine EF6(82)β cross-link	NFPLP (Bis-PL)P_4
Lysine G6(99)α_1-lysine G6(99)α_2 cross-link	Bis-(3,5-dibromosalicyl)fumarate
2,3-DPG analog	Pyridoxal 5'-phosphate
Surface, multisite	Glutaraldehyde Polyaldehydes Ring-opened dials Diimidate esters
Conjugated hemoglobin	Dextran-aldehyde Polyethylene glycol Polyoxyethylene

lysine groups provide many potential sites for modification, their large number also means that such reactions are very difficult to control.

All of the reactions currently considered to be useful in the production of hemoglobin-based blood substitutes use chemical modification at one or more of these sites (Table 5.1). Differences in the reactions are determined by the dimensions and reactivity of the cross-linking reagents. Since the function of hemoglobin in binding and releasing oxygen is intricately connected to the transition between T and R conformations, it is not surprising that the P_{50} and yield are highly variable. Even small differences among structures of the reagents can yield products with very different properties. In addition, the conditions of the reaction are very important, not only in regard to the state of ligation (i.e., oxygen saturation) but also in regard to the presence of agents or molecules that block or compete for certain reactive sites.

A further complication of these reactions is that many non-hemoglobin proteins contain reactive groups and may also be modified to produce new, potentially toxic, contaminants. It is understandable that it has been difficult to produce a "pure" modified hemoglobin for toxicity studies when most processes start with relatively crude "stroma-free" hemoglobin.

5.2 Amino-terminal Modification

5.2.1 Carbamylation

Modification of the amino-terminal groups of hemoglobin by the carbamylation reaction (Fig. 5.2) was used (1) to show that valine NA1(1)α is one of the residues involved in the alkaline Bohr effect; (2) to show the site of binding of carbon dioxide; and (3) to show that the sickling of cells containing hemoglobin S could be inhibited specifically (Manning 1981). The products of these reactions have increased oxygen affinity if the α chains are carbamylated and decreased affinity if the β chains are carbamylated.

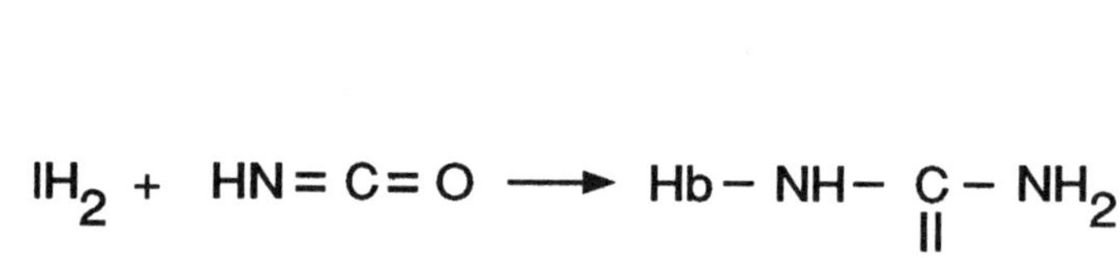

Figure 5.2. Carbamylation reaction.

The carbamylation reaction held great promise in the control of sickling, but oral administration of sodium cyanate had toxic side effects; extracorporeal carbamylation of hemoglobin and return to the patient proved to be impractical after a large effort to develop clinically useful techniques.

5.2.2 Carboxymethylation

Other modifications of the amino-terminal groups of hemoglobin also have been studied. Wendy Fantl and co-workers reasoned that a covalent adduct at the amino-terminal amino group might reduce oxygen affinity by lowering or neutralizing the net positive charge in the 2,3-DPG pocket (Fantl, Manning, et al. 1987). These workers studied

Table 5.2. Monofunctional Derivatives of Pyridoxal

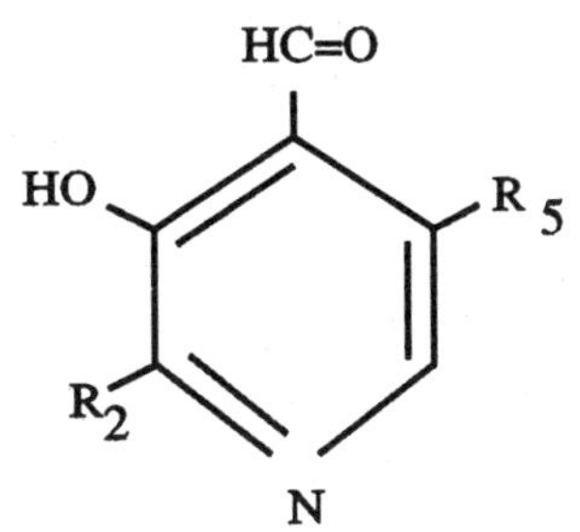

Pyridoxal	$R_2 = CH_3$; $R_5 = CH_2OH$
Pyridoxal 5' - phosphate (PLP)	$R_2 = CH_3$; $R_5 = CH_2\text{-O-}PO_3^{=}$
Pyridoxal 5' - sulfate (PLS)	$R_2 = CH_3$; $R_5 = CH2\text{-O-}SO_3^{-}$
Pyridoxal 5' - methyl - phosphonate (PMP)	$R_2 = CH_3$; $R_5 = CH_2\text{-O-P}(CH_3)O_2^{-}$
Pyridoxal 5' - phosphate monomethyl ester (PME)	$R_2 = CH_3$; $R_5 = CH_2\text{-O-P}(OCH_3)O_2^{-}$
5' - Deoxypyridoxal (DPL)	$R_2 = CH_3$; $R_5 = CH_3$
2 - Nor -2- formylpyridoxal 5' - phosphate (NFPLP)	$R_2 = CHO$; $R_5 = CH_2\text{-O-}PO_3^{=}$

Source: Benesch and Benesch (1981), with permission.

carboxymethylation with glyoxylic acid and reduction with sodium borohydride and found that the product indeed demonstrated lowered oxygen affinity and nearly intact Bohr and carbon dioxide effects (Manning et al. 1989). X-ray and nuclear magnetic resonance studies confirmed that the introduced group occupies nearly the same position as the naturally occurring carbamino group (carbon dioxide adduct) (Fantl, Donato, et al. 1987). If this modified hemoglobin could be cross-linked further to reduce its dissociation and renal excretion, it might be very attractive as a blood substitute.

5.2.3 Pyridoxal Derivatives

Benesch and Benesch showed that various aldehydes of pyridoxal (Table 5.2) could react with hemoglobin at sites that could be controlled somewhat by the state of oxygenation (Benesch et al. 1972; Benesch and Benesch 1981). They were thereby able to achieve derivatives with a wide range of functional properties. The reaction (Fig. 5.3) involves first the formation of a Schiff's base between the amino groups of hemoglobin and the aldehyde(s) of the pyridoxal compound followed by reduction of the Schiff's base with sodium borohydride to yield a covalently linked pyridoxal derivative in the form of a secondary amine.

Pyridoxal has very little reactivity with hemoglobin, but the compound with a free phosphate in the 5' position, pyridoxal 5'-phosphate (PLP), reacts specifically with the amino-terminal groups of the β-globin chain in deoxyhemoglobin. The other reagents listed in Table 5.2 (except NFPLP) react with the amino-terminal groups of α-globin chains in oxyhemoglobin.

The PLP-deoxyhemoglobin reaction was detailed by Benesch and Benesch (1981). Briefly, stripped (i.e., free of 2,3-DPG) hemoglobin in Tris buffer is deoxygenated at 10°C under nitrogen, and then is added in a molar ratio of 4.2/3 (PLP/hemoglobin). After thirty minutes, a tenfold excess of sodium borohydride is added and allowed to reduce the Schiff's base for another thirty minutes. Pure diPLP-hemoglobin (hemoglobin with both β chain amino termini modified) can be isolated by column chromatography. The structure of the product was confirmed by X-ray diffraction analysis (Arnone, Benesch, and Benesch 1977) and peptide analysis (Benesch, Benesch, and Kwong 1982), which also showed electrostatic interaction of the 5'-phosphate with the 2,3-DPG binding site, lysine EF6(82)β. Thus, this modification closely mimics the action of 2,3-DPG in stabilizing the deoxy conformation.

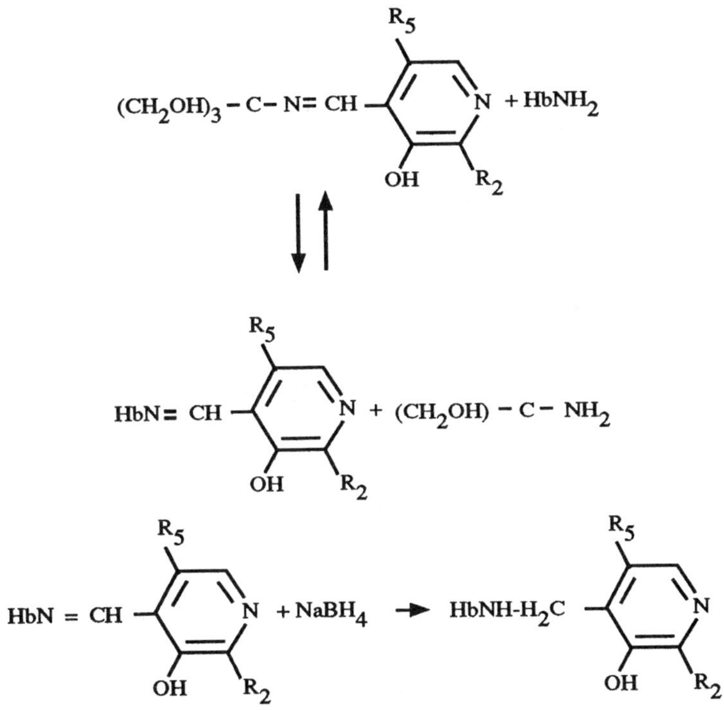

Figure 5.3. Reaction of PLP with an amino-terminal amino group of hemoglobin. The reagent is in the form of a Schiff's base with Tris, and the reaction is a transamination. The resulting unstable Schiff's base is reduced with sodium borohydride.

The oxygen affinity of the derivative was shown to be about half that of unmodified hemoglobin under similar conditions, but a degree of cooperativity was preserved. Bellelli and co-workers (1987) interpreted equilibrium and kinetic ligand binding studies on this derivative to show a perturbed R state. They believe that although the cross-link is between the two β chains, αβ dimers function independently, probably through a flexible connection.

The reaction of hemoglobin with PLP was scaled up (Sehgal et al. 1981; DeVenuto and Zegna 1983) to batches of 20 liters with yields of 70–80 percent of modified hemoglobin. Methemoglobin could be kept at a manageable level (less than 10 percent) and the material was apparently unchanged after infusion into baboons. This solution was shown to be effective in resuscitation from hemorrhagic shock (Hoyt et al. 1980; Jesch et al. 1982), but the plasma retention was thought to be too short and the COP too high to be a definitive red cell substitute (Sehgal et al. 1984; Gould, Sehgal, et al. 1986; Moss et al. 1988).

Marini and others (1989) explored the PLP reaction in the absence of Tris buffer and found that reduction of the product with cyanogen borohydride produces a lower concentration of methemoglobin than does sodium borohydride but that both reagents yield a heterogeneous mixture of products (Fig. 5.4). Others (Sekuguchi et al. 1985; McGarrity, Er,

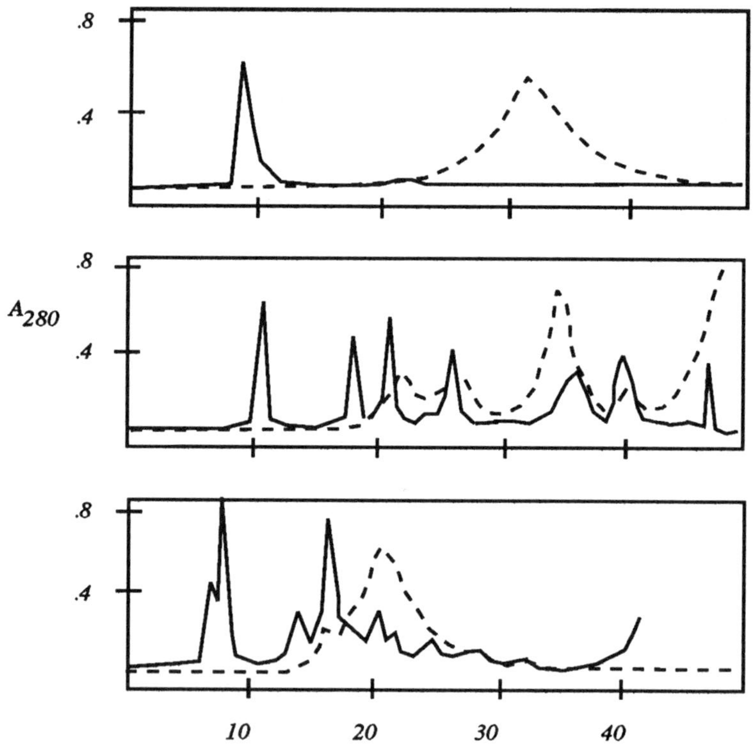

Figure 5.4. Analytical chromatograms of the reaction products of hemoglobin A_0 with PLP (1 mol per mol heme). (*Top*) Unreduced PLP-Hb; (*Middle*) PLP-Hb reduced in the oxy form with four molar equivalents of sodium borohydride; (*Bottom*) PLP-Hb reduced with four molar equivalents of sodium cyanoborohydride. The *dashed lines* represent radioactivity. *Source*: Marini et al. (1989), with permission.

Nightingale, and Hsia 1987) have also found heterogeneity of products and reported that the P_{50} decreased on storage if the temperature is above 4°C. Some of the heterogeneity can be explained by exchange of αβ subunits (Menu et al. 1987).

Thus, the large-scale preparation of pyridoxylated hemoglobin seems to result in mixtures of reaction products. These probably represent modifications at either or both α and β amino-terminal residues as well as surface lysines. A partial characterization of this mixture has been carried out (McGarrity, Er, and Hsia 1987). The real question is whether such heterogeneity should be permitted in a solution prepared for use in humans, and there is as yet no definite answer. If the solutions have little or no toxicity, then perhaps heterogeneity can be tolerated. But if they are toxic the presence of multiple components will increase the difficulty in determining mechanisms.

5.2.4 Acetaldehyde

Acetaldehyde was found to have a slightly different reaction mechanism with hemoglobin (San George and Hoberman 1986). Although this reagent does react with surface lysines under some conditions, the principal products are derivatives of the amino-terminal groups, both of the α and β chains. These products are not reduced with sodium borohydride and therefore do not involve an intermediate Schiff's base. Instead, a stable cyclic imidazolidinone derivative is formed. This reaction has not been developed further for use as a red cell substitute.

5.2.5 Lysine EF6(82)β Modification

An interesting modification of human hemoglobin was reported by Bucci and co-workers which they called a pseudocross-link (Bucci, Razynska, Urbaitis, and Fronticelli 1989). In this reaction, hemoglobin is reacted with mono-(3,5-dibromosalicyl)-fumarate in oxygenated conditions. The product is specifically acylated at lysine EF6(82)β, in about 70 percent yield. Cooperativity is reduced somewhat (Hill coefficient of 2.0), but the P_{50} under physiologic conditions is 25 torr, and carbon dioxide binding is intact since the sites for carbon dioxide binding are unaffected. Bucci and co-workers found that the tetramer-dimer dissociation is retarded, possibly by stabilization at the ββ interface (Bucci, Fronticelli, Razynska, and Urbaitis 1989). The resulting plasma retention half-time in the rat is also prolonged by about fourfold, compared with unmodified hemoglobin. This modification represents a new class of reactions that have potential for specificity and high yield.

5.3 Valine NA1(1)β_1 - Lysine EF6(82)β_2 Cross-link

5.3.1 2-Nor-2-formylpyridoxal 5'-Phosphate

2-Nor-2-formylpyridoxal 5'-phosphate (NFPLP, Table 5.2) is of special interest because it contains two reactive aldehyde groups. Thus, as shown in Figure 5.5, it reacts at two sites, the amino-terminal group of one β chain and the lysine 82 of the other (Benesch et al. 1975; Arnone, Benesch, and Benesch 1977). Thus, with one modification reaction, this reagent both reduces the oxygen affinity of native hemoglobin and prevents its dissociation into αβ dimers.

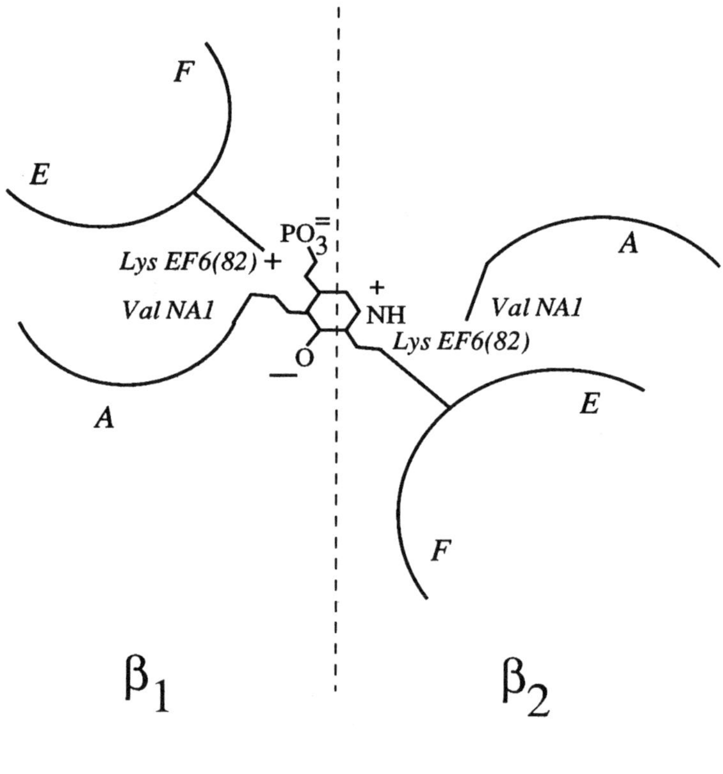

Figure 5.5. Reaction of NFPLP with hemoglobin. *Source:* adapted from Benesch and Benesch (1981).

This derivative has been studied extensively. Because dimerization is prevented, NFPLP is not eliminated in the urine (Sloviter et al. 1981;

Triner et al. 1983; Keipert et al. 1988), and its plasma retention is at least three times that of either unmodified hemoglobin (Sloviter et al. 1981) or pyridoxylated hemoglobin (Bleeker et al. 1986). Its pattern of tissue distribution and elimination has been documented in detail (Keipert and Triner 1989; Keipert et al. 1989; Bleeker et al. 1989). Of particular interest is the fact that accumulation of this derivative in the kidney is much reduced as compared with unmodified hemoglobin (Bleeker et al. 1989). Its oxygen affinity under physiologic conditions is about 47 torr; it retains cooperativity; and when used to perfuse isolated organs, it supports a higher tissue oxygen tension in the rabbit heart (Benesch et al. 1984) and rat liver (VanderPlas et al. 1986; Bakker, Bleeker and VanderPlas 1986).

Although the 60–80 percent yield of the NFPLP product would seem satisfactory (VanderPlas, Damm, and Bakker 1987), the main drawback seems to be the difficulty in preparation of the reagent (Benesch and Benesch 1981). However, Bakker and co-workers in the Netherlands (Bakker, Bleeker, and VanderPlas 1986; VanderPlas, Damm, and Bakker 1987; VanderPlas et al. 1986; Bleeker et al. 1986, 1989) have sustained a major effort to develop this derivative as a blood substitute.

5.3.2 Bis-pyridoxal Tetraphosphate

A second class of bifunctional reagents (Table 5.3) was described by Benesch and Kwong (1988). These involve two pyridoxal groups linked by phosphate of different lengths.

As shown in Table 5.3, the yield of intramolecularly cross-linked hemoglobin increases dramatically with increasing length of the phosphate backbone. Benesch and Kwong (1988) believe the site of reaction of (bis-PL)P_4 is between the amino terminal amino-group of one β chain and the lysine 82 of the other β chain, as is the case with NFPLP. However, the distance between these two residues is only 11Å, and the reagent is much longer. Therefore the authors conclude that the cross-linker must fold back upon itself to form a "stacked" pyridine ring conformation.

Hemoglobin modified with this reagent was studied further by Keipert and others (Keipert, Aderiran, Kwong, and Benesch 1989) who showed that its P_{50} is 31 torr (pH 7.4, PCO_2 40 torr, 37°C), with a Bohr effect about half that of unmodified hemoglobin. Its plasma retention is prolonged threefold in the rat, and there was no apparent toxicity in screening studies. These results suggest its utility as a blood substitute. A

Table 5.3. Bis-Pyridoxal Polyphosphates

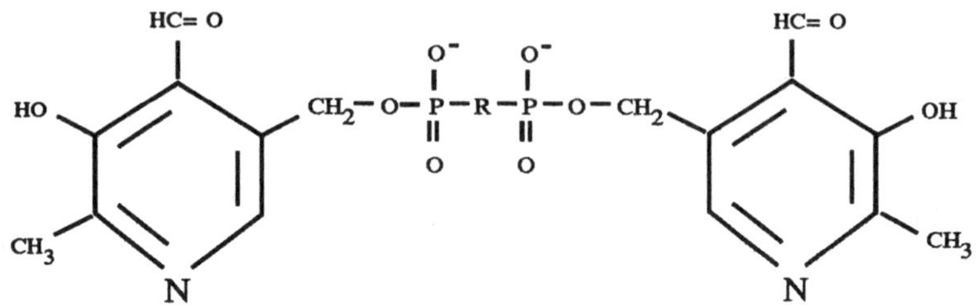

Abbreviation	R	% Tetramer
(Bis-PL)P_2	Oxygen	16
(Bis-PL)P_3	Orthophosphate	18
(Bis-PL)P_4	Pyrophosphate	68
CH_2-(bis-PL)P_4	Methylene diphosphate	53
Fructose (bis-PL)P_4	Fructose 1,6-diphosphate	41
PLP-DPG-PLP	2,3-Diphosphoglycerate	70

Source: Benesch and Kwong (1988), with permission

great advantage of (bis-PL)P_4 is that its synthesis is much simpler than that for NFPLP. It is likely therefore that this derivative may be studied in laboratories that do not have highly specialized equipment for the industrial production of modified hemoglobin (Winslow 1989).

5.3.3 Other 2,3-Diphosphoglycerate Pocket Cross-linkers

The reactivity of the valine NA1(1)α-lysine EF6(82)β residues in the 2,3-DPG pocket shown by NFPLP and (bis-PL)P_4 has stimulated the search for other reagents that react similarly but with potential for greater efficiency and scaleup. Richard Jones and co-workers (1989) reported on the systematic study of four different dicarboxylic acid derivatives, cross-linked in both oxygenated and deoxygenated conditions. Each of these derivatives presents unique problems in purification, and proof of the sites of reaction is tedious. However, if safety and efficacy of internally cross-linked hemoglobin tetramers with suitable oxygen affinity can be demonstrated using the model derivatives made with NFPLP and (bis-PL)P_4, then development of these alternatives will surely advance quickly.

5.4 Lysine G6(99)α_1 - Lysine G6(99)α_2 Cross-link

Joseph Walder and co-workers described a class of bifunctional reagents that could cross-link human hemoglobin in the oxy form (Zaugg, King, and Klotz 1975; Walder et al. 1979; Walder, Walder, and Arnone 1980; Wood et al. 1981). The derivatives were thought to have potential in preventing sickling in patients with sickle-cell anemia because they increased the oxygen affinity of native hemoglobin. When the cross-linking reaction was carried out in the oxy form, the site of reaction was shown to be between lysine EF6(82)β_1 and lysine EF6(82)β_2 (Walder, Walder, and Arnone 1980).

Tye and co-workers (1983) studied the usefulness of one of the reagents, bis(3,5-dibromosalicyl)fumarate (DBBF), in the production of a blood substitute and reported their results in 1982 at an international symposium on blood substitutes which was held in San Francisco. One of Tye's colleagues, Francisco Medina, had discovered that if the cross-linking reaction was carried out under anaerobic conditions, the product had reduced, rather than increased, oxygen affinity. Unfortunately, Tye et al. assigned the site of substitution incorrectly, believing it to cross-link the lysine EF6(82)β-valine NA1(1)α residues as NFPLP did, but the results were very encouraging because they showed promise that a single modification could achieve the dual goals of reduced oxygen affinity and restricted tetramer-dimer dissociation.

The U.S. Army chose to develop the reagent DBBF further (under contract to Baxter Healthcare Corp.) because of the potential simplicity of its reaction with hemoglobin and the possibility of isolating single components for the careful study of toxicity. Chatterjee et al. (1986) showed subsequently that the site of cross-linking in DBBF-modified hemoglobin is between lysine G6(99)α_1 and lysine G6(99)α_2 (Fig. 5.6), and Snyder et al. (1987) confirmed the earlier work of Tye et al. This product was called $\alpha\alpha$-hemoglobin ($\alpha\alpha$-Hb).

The product was formulated in Ringer's lactate. P_{50} is 28.0 torr; Hill's parameter, 2.2; and the Bohr effect is reduced (Vandegriff et al. 1989). Plasma retention is increased, and the product appears to be less heterogeneous than some of the other derivatives currently under study.

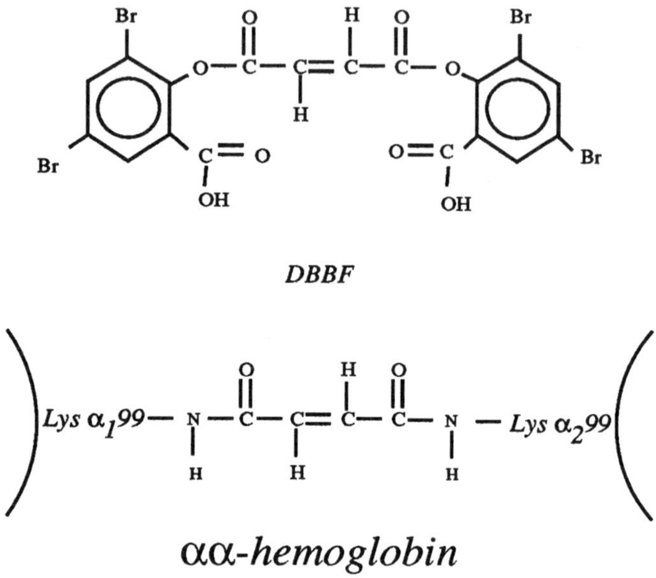

Figure 5.6. Reaction of bis(3,5-dibromosalicyl)fumarate with hemoglobin.

An interesting property of DBBF-hemoglobin is its increased thermal stability (Table 5.4). Olsen and co-workers (Yang and Olsen 1988; White and Olsen 1987) showed that human hemoglobin, cross-linked in the oxy state, had increased stability to heat, especially in the liganded (CO) form. Estep and others took advantage of this property to achieve both a partial purification of the crude reaction mixture after cross linking, and inactivation of viruses in the final product (Estep et al. 1988; Estep et al. 1989).

Table 5.4. Thermal Stability of Hemoglobin Cross-linked with DBBF

	T_m	
	Native	Cross-linked
Met A	44.3	57.9
CN-met A	55.5	53.6
Carboxyhemoglobin A	54.9	63.9

Source: data from Yang and Olsen (1988).
Note: T_m is the transition temperature (^{o}C) at which half of the protein is denatured, measured optically at 280 nm.

5.5 Surface, Multisite Reagents

The addition of reactive groups to the surface of hemoglobin has been one of the most popular modifications because it results in large aggregates of molecules. These aggregates have the advantage of prolonging the intravascular retention time, but their disadvantage is that the extent of polymerization may be difficult to control as well as nonspecific. The reagents are polyfunctional aldehydes, of which glutaraldehyde is the prime example (Fig. 5.7).

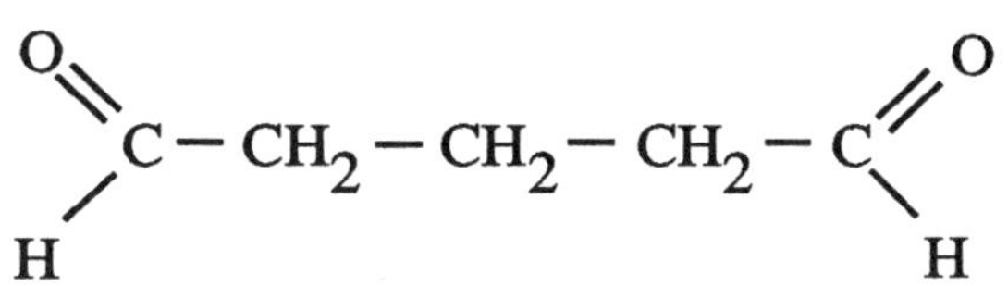

Figure 5.7. Structure of glutaraldehyde.

5.5.1 Glutaraldehyde

Gould et al. (1980) reported polymerization of pyridoxylated human hemoglobin with glutaraldehyde. Shortly thereafter, DeVenuto and Zegna (1981) also reported preparation of this derivative, and in the years that followed, this "polyhemoglobin" was studied intensively. Although many research groups have contributed to the information about this product, the team at Michael Reese Hospital in Chicago has commercialized it to the extent that limited clinical trials have been carried out in humans. Their process begins with pyridoxylated hemoglobin (14–16 g/dl) that is then polymerized with a 12.5 percent solution of glutaraldehyde. When the COP of the reaction mixture reaches normal values (20–25 torr), the reaction is "quenched" by the addition of 1.3 M/l lysine. The resulting product has a distribution of molecular masses from 120,000 to 600,000 daltons. The product has a P_{50} of 16 torr, a Bohr effect reduced by about half, and a Hill coefficient of 1.7. The viscosity is 4.5 centipoise, compared with 1.8 for unpolymerized hemoglobin. The Michael Reese team also reported that these solutions had no effect on coagulation, as measured by the prothrombin or partial thromboplastin times.

As shown in Table 5.5, at equivalent COP, the polymerized solution has a higher hemoglobin concentration and therefore can carry more oxygen. Subsequent physiologic studies carried out by this group (Sehgal, et al. 1984; Gould, Rosen, Sehgal, Sehgal, and Moss 1986) showed that the product transports oxygen as expected and that the reduced P_{50} did not diminish its usefulness (Rosen et al. 1986). The plasma half-life of this product in baboons was remarkably prolonged, to 46.2 hours, compared with 5.9 hours for PLP-hemoglobin (Sehgal et al. 1984).

The procedure used by DeVenuto and Zegna (1983) differed mainly in that the starting material was "crystallized" hemoglobin (DeVenuto, Zuck, Zegna, and Moores 1977; DeVenuto, Zegna, and Busse 1979). In their polymerization procedure, a 7/1 molar ratio glutaraldehyde to hemoglobin was used, with a hemoglobin solution of 14 g/dl concentration. Their description did not include quenching the reaction as did that of Sehgal et al. (1984). DeVenuto and Zegna (1982) showed that the effects of PLP and glutaraldehyde on oxygen affinity are opposed: glutaraldehyde decreases P_{50}, but PLP increases it. DeVenuto and his coworkers (1982) and their colleagues then reported a series of studies in a variety of animals and showed that their product could support life at zero hematocrit in rats and that its renal toxicity was minimal (Friedman et al. 1984). Marks later carried out an optimization study for the conditions of the reactions with PLP and glutaraldehyde and found considerable batch-to-batch variability (Marks et al. 1988).

Table 5.5. Properties of Pyridoxylated, Polymerized Hemoglobin (PLP-polyHb)

Hemoglobin concentration	12 to 14 g/dl
Methemoglobin	<5 percent
Molecular weight	64,000 to 400,000
Mean molecular mass	150,000
P_{50}	18.2 torr
n (Hill's parameter)	1.5 to 2.2
Bohr factor	- 0.12 to - 0.25
Colloid osmotic pressure	20 to 25 mm Hg
Viscosity	1.9 to 2.2 cp
Endotoxin	<0.625 EU/ml
Rabbit pyrogen test	Pass

Source: data from Sehgal et al. (1980).

Moore (Moore, Ledford, and Tillotson 1986), Marini et al. (1990), Agostoni et al. (1987), and Hsia (1989) have all reexamined the products of the glutaraldehyde reaction of pyridoxylated hemoglobin and found extreme heterogeneity (Fig. 5.8). They showed that the products are unstable on storage at $4^{o}C$; rearrangements of polymeric species occur so that it is difficult to prepare a predictably modified species. This heterogeneity and instability are regarded as serious drawbacks of the product because reactions with plasma proteins in vivo would be impossible to predict, and toxicity would be difficult to understand. Agostoni et al. (1987) raised the particular concern that the low molecular weight material might be lost preferentially through the kidneys, leaving the inherently more unstable polymers, which have less favorable oxygen transport properties.

Glutaraldehyde treatment of hemoglobin has the effect of making the tetrameric structure of the molecule more rigid. Indeed, it seems that the more highly modified (polymerized), the more rigid hemoglobin molecules become, as reflected in increasing oxygen affinity and decreasing cooperativity. Studies using the very sensitive Mössbaur technique (Guillochon et al. 1986) have shown that glutaraldehyde-treated hemoglobin has an increased rate of autooxidation and increased thermal stability. These properties could be explained by a weakening of the heme-globin linkage (see Chapter 3).

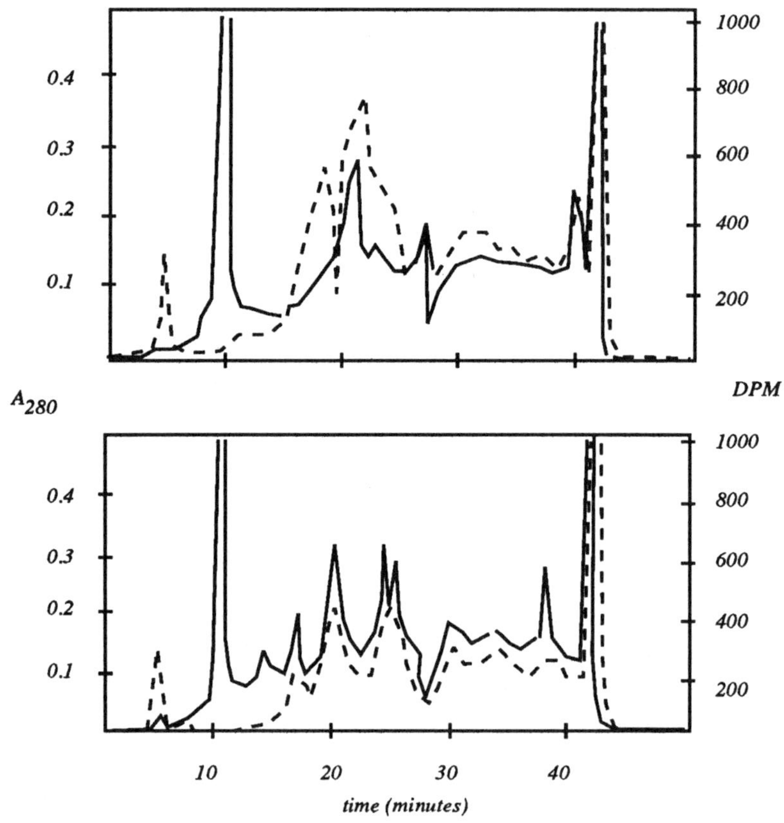

Figure 5.8. Products of glutaraldehyde reaction with hemoglobin. *Dashed line* represents radioactivity. *Source:* Marini et al. (1990), with permission.

The heterogeneity of the glutaraldehyde product could make toxicology studies difficult. The heterogeneity is a result of chemical bonds that tend to rearrange; thus, it is conceivable that glutaraldehyde could "leach" out of the protein. Glutaraldehyde itself is known to leach out of materials used for prosthetic devices (Gendler, Gendler, and Nimni 1984; McPherson, Sawamura, and Armstrong 1986). It is used as a tissue fixative and even small amounts of free glutaraldehyde have been found to have cytotoxic activity (Speer et al. 1980).

5.5.2 Other Polyaldehydes

A number of dialdehyde reagents can be prepared by oxidizing the ring structures of sugars or nucleotides (Scannon 1982) (Fig. 5.9). These reagents can react with hemoglobin at any of its amino groups and therefore form a variety of modifications including intramolecular and intermolecular links. One example of this type of modification, opening the ring of inositol tetraphosphate, is discussed below. Another, described by Greenburg and Maffuid (Greenburg and Maffuid 1983) involves the opening of the pyridine ring of ATP. Hemoglobin so modified (ATP-hemoglobin) was reported by Greenburg and Maffuid to have an elevated P_{50} and normal cooperativity.

Scannon (1982) reported that ATP-hemoglobin had relatively unchanged P_{50}, but Hsia et al. (1986) optimized the reaction conditions and

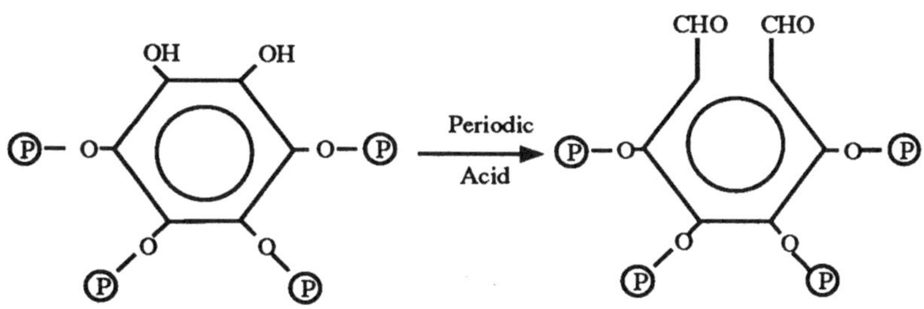

Figure 5.9. Preparation of dialdehyde by oxidation of inositol hexaphosphate (IHP) with vicinyl hydroxyls. *Source*: adapted from Wong (1988).

were able to produce a preparation with markedly reduced affinity. McGarrity, Nightingale, and Hsia (1987) isolated five fractions from a reaction mixture and found their P_{50} values to range from 8 to 38 torr, most with little cooperativity. These results are consistent with those found with other polyfunctional reagents that react on the surface of hemoglobin, and the extreme heterogeneity should not be surprising with regard to either species present or their functional properties.

5.6 Diimidate Esters

Diimidate esters are bifunctional reagents that have been used in cross-linking a variety of proteins, including hemoglobin. A typical reaction is shown in Figure 5.10, where a lysyl ε-amino group reacts with the ester. The reagent is specific for surface ε-amino groups and forms polymers of varying size. One of the advantages of the reaction is that it replaces the $-NH_3^+$ group with a $=NH_2^+$ group, so the overall charge is changed very little. The product reported by Mok, Chen and Mazur (1975) had thirty of the forty-four surface lysyl residues modified and had a molecular mass ranging from 68,000 to 600,000 daltons. Intravascular retention time was increased by about fourfold in rabbits.

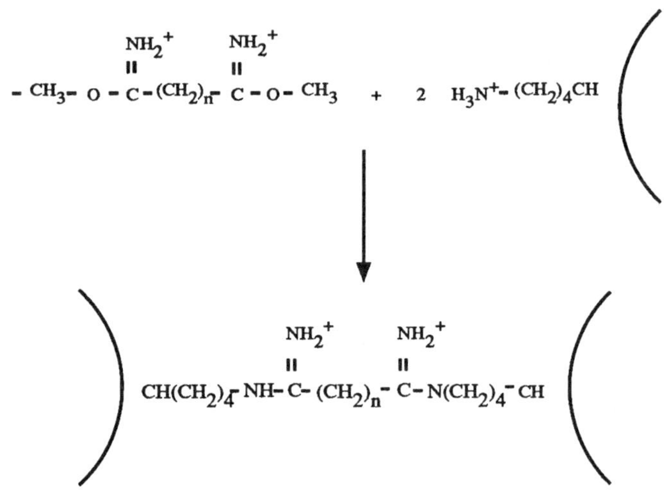

Figure 5.10. Reaction of lysyl ε-amino group with diimidate esters. n = 1 for malonimidate, n = 4 for adipimidate, n = 6 for suberimidate, and n = 8 for sebacimidate. *Source*: adapted from Mok, Chen, and Mazur (1975).

5.7 Conjugated Hemoglobin

An alternative approach to prolongation of the plasma retention is to conjugate hemoglobin to a larger molecule. Wong and his co-workers were the first to exploit this concept, coupling hemoglobin to dextran (Tam, Blumenstein, and Wong 1976; Chang and Wong 1977; Blumenstein et al. 1978; Tam, Blumenstein, and Wong 1978).

The coupling reaction is carried out using a lysate of human red cells and bromodextran, molecular weight 20,000. This product was shown to support life in the absence of red cells in dogs (Chang and Wong 1977; Blumenstein et al. 1978; Tam, Blumenstein, and Wong 1978) and cats (Humphries et al. 1981), and it did not appear to be immunogenic (Cunnington et al. 1981). But because the oxygen affinity of dextran-hemoglobin was essentially that of hemoglobin, Wong modified it further by covalently linking an analog of inositol hexaphosphate (Wong 1988; Wu, Porter and Wong 1989). This new derivative had a P_{50} of 55 torr, compared with 23 torr for dextran-hemoglobin, and the oxygenation curve was cooperative. The conjugated, right-shifted product was used to show that the modifications resulted in a reduction in renal toxicity of unpurified hemoglobin (Tam and Wong 1988).

Hemoglobin also can be conjugated to other synthetic polymers such as inulin (Iwasaki, Ajisaka, and Iwashita 1983), polyvinylpyrrolidone (Schmidt 1979), and polyethylene glycol (Ajisaka and Iwashita 1980; Leonard and Dellacherie 1984). One of the most studied of these conjugates is pyridoxylated hemoglobin-polyoxyethylene (PHP-Hb) (Ajisaka and Iwashita 1980). PHP-Hb has a molecular mass of about 90,000 daltons, a P_{50} of about 22 torr, compared with 15 torr for hemoglobin under the same conditions, but has reduced cooperativity (Matsushita et al. 1988). The plasma retention half-life in dogs is about thirty-six hours, and it apparently causes no renal, hepatic, or coagulation toxicity. Histologic examination of the lungs and spleen of transfused dogs at two weeks and later showed no abnormalities (Matsushita et al. 1988).

5.8 Starting Material and Purification

If toxicity of modified hemoglobin solutions were not a problem, the purity of starting material might be irrelevant. Thus, Rabiner's method (Rabiner et al. 1967) for the filtration purification of hemoglobin was thought to be a major advance over centrifugation methods (Brown and Dale 1936; Hamilton, Farr, Hiller, and VanSlyke 1947). However, hemoglobin prepared in this way caused unwanted reactions in human recipients (Savitsky et al. 1978). DeVenuto and co-workers (1977) described a subsequent method, which they called "crystallization." They found it to show fewer toxic effects in animals (DeVenuto et al. 1977) but batch-to-batch reproducibility was uneven (Moore, Ledford, and Tillotson 1986). Thus, each new advance in the purification of hemoglobin has offered the hope of eliminating toxicity, only to be followed by the discovery of new or continued difficulties. Our approach has been to use only the most rigorously purified starting material for producing cross-linked hemoglobins (Christensen et al. 1988).

Hemoglobin is provided by the red cell in highly purified form. However, the red cell contains many enzymes and other proteins, and red cell membranes contain many components that could potentially cause toxicity problems. In addition, the chemical modification reactions discussed above are not specific for hemoglobin and may modify other proteins as well. Indeed, multifunctional reagents could actually couple hemoglobin to some of these nonhemoglobin proteins.

The method used in our laboratory involves high-pressure liquid chromatography (HPLC) purification of red cell lysates. The effectiveness of this procedure is illustrated in Table 5.6, which shows various enzymatic activities at various stages of purification.

Using a preparative HPLC apparatus, it is possible to prepare more than 60 g of protein in a single run. This material contains less than one percent methemoglobin and is sterile and endotoxin free. It can be stored

Table 5.6. Enzymatic Activity of Hemoglobin Solutions

Enzyme	RBC (IU/gHb)	SFH (IU/gHb)	HbA_o (IU/gHb)
Hexokinase	1.2	0.7	0
Triosephosphate isomerase	2,100	1,042	0
Glyceraldehyde-3-phosphate dehydrogenase	226	56	0
Lactate dehydrogenase	200	197	0
Phosphoglycerate kinase	320	195	0
Glucose-6-phosphate dehydrogenase	8.3	0.9	0
Glutathione reductase	7.2	5.1	0
Glutathione peroxidase	31	5.8	Trace
NADPH diaphorase	3.4	Trace	Trace
Glutamate-oxalacetate transaminase	3.0	1.4	0
Adenosine deaminase	1.1	Trace	0

Source: data from Christensen et al. (1988).

frozen indefinitely without excessive oxidation. Of particular importance is that the level of phosphate is undetectable by atomic absorption analysis. Perfusion of this material in the isolated rabbit heart shows that it is free of vasoconstrictor activity (Macdonald et al. 1989). Our group feels strongly that until all toxic effects of hemoglobin solutions are understood completely, material of the highest possible purity should be used for modification reactions.

5.9 The Supply of Raw Materials

5.9.1 Outdated Human Blood

If clinical efficacy and safety of hemoglobin solutions can be shown, the demand for product would soon outstrip the supply of outdated human blood. As Table 5.7 shows, about 12 million units of blood are used in the United States each year, and only about 500,000 outdate. If a completely safe and efficacious product were available, perhaps the use of human blood could be reduced by as much as 50 percent because its primary use currently is in intraoperative and emergency settings. If the same number of units are drawn each year, the number available for use in production of blood substitutes could approach 6 million. Assuming a 50 percent overall production yield, 3 million units of hemoglobin solution could be produced, but these would need to satisfy the requirements for 6 million units of blood!

Thus, collection of additional units of blood would be necessary to serve as raw material for a product that is likely to be more expensive than blood itself. This proposal would be feasible only if the product could be demonstrated unequivocally to be superior to blood in certain clinical applications.

Table 5.7. Usage of Blood in the United States

Units collected	12,500,000
Units used	12,000,000
Available (outdated)	500,000

Source: data from National Institutes of Health Consensus Conference (1988).

How likely is it that hemoglobin solutions are clinically better than cellular blood products? It may be that the superior ratio of oxygen content to viscosity of hemoglobin solution could actually make them superior in perfusion or reperfusion applications: shock/resuscitation, organ perfusion and preservation, and angioplasty. Intraoperative hemodilution might also be better served with a hemoglobin solution. But any toxicity of hemoglobin solutions would prompt clinicians to use blood or red cells if they were available. The military use of hemoglobin solutions would seem the most certain because in time of need red cells may simply not be available, and frontline use of hemoglobin would offer advantages over frozen blood.

In the final analysis it would seem at this point unlikely that freshly drawn blood would be diverted for use in the manufacture of hemoglobin solutions in significant quantity or that acquisition from human donors could be increased for this purpose. An exception to this conclusion might be in the military, wherein a "captive" pool of donors exists.

5.9.2 Bovine Hemoglobin

One solution to the supply problem is to use as a starting material blood from nonhuman sources. Bovine hemoglobin, for example, is being developed by some. To satisfy the requirements for 6 million units per year, about 150,000 cows would need to be killed. This is based on 40 units per cow and 100 percent efficiency of production. It would probably be possible for a company to obtain large amounts of bovine blood from commercial sources. The ultimate success of bovine hemoglobin (or any other product), however, will depend on demonstration of its safety, not its supply.

Currently the FDA is very concerned about bovine products of all types because of the bovine spongiform encephalitis virus, identified in cows in Europe (Cherfas 1990). Related to the scrapie organism, this virus presents a potential problem with bovine hemoglobin that could be generalized to other animals. In fact, the virus has been detected in mammals other than cows in North America. It has proven to be especially resistant to heat treatment.

Bovine hemoglobin has certain desirable qualities for use as a blood substitute. Among them is its lower oxygen affinity than human hemoglobin's, under conditions found in the red cell, because of its greater sensitivity to anions (Bunn, 1971; Feola et al. 1983; Fronticelli, Bucci, and Orth 1984; Fronticelli et al. 1986). Thus, instead of regulation by 2,3-DPG, as is the case with human hemoglobin, bovine hemoglobin oxygen affinity is regulated by chloride ion.

Fronticelli et al. (1986) cross-linked bovine hemoglobin with the bifunctional reagent DBBF to obtain a product with a P_{50} in excess of 40 torr under physiologic conditions. Although the reaction mixture was somewhat heterogeneous, no uncross-linked material was detected by sedimentation velocity analysis, and the plasma retention in rats was prolonged tenfold compared with unmodified hemoglobin.

DeVenuto (1988) also studied modified bovine hemoglobin. He found that the pyridoxylation reaction raises the P_{50} from 28.5 to 38.0 torr, and glutaraldehyde polymerization drops the P_{50} to 18 torr. The polymerized material had essentially the same plasma retention time as human hemoglobin modified in the same way, and rats could also be supported at zero hematocrit.

5.9.3 Recombinant Hemoglobin

An alternative and novel source of hemoglobin for modification is from microorganisms whose genome has been modified to contain globin genes, recombinant hemoglobin (rHb). Major strides have been made in this approach in recent years, and it is now possible to express both human α and β globin chains in *E.coli* (Hoffman et al. 1990).

There are several problems with this approach. First, the yield is quite low using the current technology. The best yield that has been reported to date is about 0.1 g per liter of culture. Since 1 unit of blood (500 ml) contains about 15 g per liter of hemoglobin, a total of 75 g of hemoglobin equal to 750 liters of cell culture would be needed. To satisfy the 6 million unit requirement, 6 million units x 0.5 l x 750 = 2.25 billion liters of cell culture would be required! In the future it might be possible to express hemoglobin genes in higher organisms; synthesis of functional human hemoglobin has already been reported in mice (Behringer et al. 1989).

Another problem of rHb production is its purity. The product would need to be separated from media components and other microorganism products. Endotoxin contamination could be a serious problem for *Escherichia coli* products, and low yield is an additional problem in yeast systems. Thus, the state of the microbe-expressed hemoglobin efforts at this time can be summarized as in need of a dramatic breakthrough in scaleup technology and improved yields. Nevertheless, this source would appear to be the ultimate solution to the supply problem if these obstacles can be overcome.

Finally, this approach is valid only if hemoglobin or some derivative is shown to be safe for human use. Recombinant hemoglobin will do little to solve the significant remaining toxicity problems except as a source for well-characterized hemoglobin molecules.

Chapter 6

The Efficacy of Hemoglobin-based Red Cell Substitutes

It is intuitively apparent that a red cell replacement solution should carry as much oxygen as possible. Indeed, this assumption has sustained the effort to develop a hemoglobin-containing blood substitute for more than fifty years. It would seem that solid experimental proof of the assumption would be relatively easy to establish; however, the question of efficacy is more complex than it seems at first glance. In fact, establishing efficacy actually requires answers to several questions. *Can* oxygen-carrying solutions work? *Will* they work in specific clinical situations? Can they be made *available* for use? Are they *worth* using (i.e., superior to other forms of therapy)?

Answers are not available for all of these questions. The greatest impediment to establishing efficacy fully for hemoglobin-based red cell substitutes has been the lack of high-quality, well-characterized, reproducibly prepared products for testing. Early efficacy studies were conducted with relatively crude materials that gave results that were difficult to repeat and confirm. Only when Rabiner et al. (1967) demonstrated that removal of red blood cell stroma decreased toxicity was awareness of the importance of this problem appreciated. Thus, the issues of modification, production, and toxicity are intimately connected to efficacy.

Furthermore, the question of efficacy of hemoglobin solutions must be qualified immediately by a statement of what it is intended to be efficacious *for*. Hemoglobin solutions have two physiologically important properties: colloid osmotic pressure (COP) and oxygen transport. Both of these are important in the trauma setting: COP maintains intravascular volume, and oxygen is transported to ischemic tissue. Both are essential to successful resuscitation, but there are other applications that do not require colloid. Many solutions already in clinical use provide colloid; albumin and dextran, for example, do. It is the oxygen transport function of hemoglobin which makes it unique.

6.1 Early Studies

Several early studies showed that hemoglobin solutions transport oxygen. Salaskin and Kriwsky (1931) were the first to use hemoglobin added to Ringer-Locke solution to perfuse a liver. They showed that urea could be synthesized by the organ when given ammonium carbonate as substrate. Urea was not produced when the perfusion solution was Ringer-Locke solution alone. Soon thereafter, Amberson and his co-workers (Amberson and Höber 1932; Amberson et al. 1933) extended these observations to show that even more complex physiologic functions could be preserved in isolated salivary glands with the use of hemoglobin-Ringer's solution.

In discussing physiologic saline and other blood substitutes, Amberson wrote, "It is impossible to maintain life in the whole mammalian body after the complete replacement of the normal blood with any salt solution" (Amberson 1937, 49). He noted that after administration of saline to a severely hemorrhaged animal, the blood pressure increase lasts only for a few minutes because of shifts of intravascular fluid. Other similar colloid-lacking solutions such as lactate, Ringer's glucose solution, and urea solution are also useful only for a few minutes. He went on, "It is reasonable to expect, therefore, that when all other organic constituents are removed, dissolved hemoglobin will be able to confer, upon an otherwise synthetic solution, an ability to function effectively as a substitute for whole blood" (Amberson 1937, 56–57). He considered the two properties of hemoglobin, COP and oxygen-carrying capacity, to be equally important.

In 1933 Amberson and his colleagues reported complete exchange transfusions in cats with hemoglobin-containing Ringer's lactate (Amberson et al. 1933). They wrote, "After the removal of the normal blood under ether anesthesia the animals may regain consciousness and exhibit an essentially normal behavior for several hours. Our best experiments of this type have been with cats. They are able to walk, run, see and hear. They are able to jump to the floor from a considerable height, judge distances correctly and make their way about in a normal manner. All postural and equilibratory reflexes appear to be normal. When dropped upside down they land on their feet." Although these animals fared well immediately after the exchange, "such animals finally die, after five or six hours, not because the hemoglobin is unable to carry on its function, but because it leaves the blood stream with much greater ease than do the normal plasma proteins" (Amberson et al. 1933, 107).

Much of the early work on the biologic effects of hemoglobin-containing solutions was carried out between 1934 and 1949 by Amberson and his colleagues. The solution they used for their animal studies was called hemoglobin-Ringer's because it consisted essentially of Ringer's solution to which was added bovine hemoglobin. In their most successful experiments they added, to 1 liter of solution, the hemoglobin from up to 500 ml of washed and hemolyzed bovine red cells (Table 6.1).

Fresh beef blood was defibrinated by agitation, and the serum was removed. The red cells were washed twice in Ringer-Locke solution. The red cells (500 ml) were then added to 490 ml of distilled water, chilled to $5^{o}C$, and allowed to stand for 15 minutes. The other ingredients listed in Table 6.1 were then added as solid reagents, and the stromata were removed by "long centrifugation." The composition of the final solution is given in Table 6.1.

Table 6.1. Composition and Properties of Hemoglobin-Ringer's

Composition	
Hemoglobin	130–140 g/liter
Na^{+}	3.70 g/liter
K^{+}	0.36 g/liter
Ca^{2+}	0.10 g/liter
Cl^{-}	4.95 g/liter
PO_4^{3-}	0.50 g/liter
HCO_3^{-}	1.00–1.40 g/liter
Properties	
COP	55–60 torr
pH ($38^{o}C$)	7.3–7.4
O_2 content	17–19 vol %
CO_2 content	15–20 vol %
	Isotonic

Source: data from Amberson et al. (1934–35).

A significant milestone in establishing efficacy occurred when a complete exchange transfusion was carried out in cats using hemoglobin-

Ringer's solution (Mulder et al. 1934). Figure 6.1 shows that respiratory activity and the rate of oxygen consumption of the animal were unchanged even at zero hematocrit. This experiment showed unequivocally that hemoglobin-Ringer's transports oxygen to respiring tissues, and, although not designed to simulate a realistic clinical application, this experiment has been cited by current workers (Moss et al. 1988) as establishing efficacy of cell-free hemoglobin solutions.

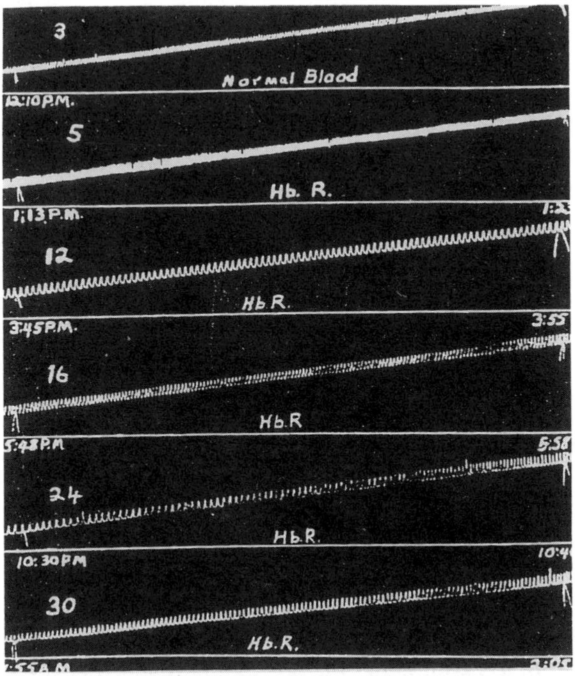

Figure 6.1. Original recording of the respiratory movements of a cat during exchange transfusion with hemoglobin-Ringer's solution. The *top panel (3)* is the control. Subsequent panels were recorded after the exchange. *Source:* Mulder et al. (1934), copyright © 1934. Reprinted by permission of Wiley-Liss, a division of John Wiley and Sons, Inc.

A 1940 study (Buttle, Kekwick, and Schweitzer 1940) compared hemoglobin solutions with other standard therapies of the time and pointed out many of the pitfalls of such efficacy studies. Buttle and his coworkers established a standard (50 percent) lethal hemorrhage in anesthetized cats. The result was an arterial blood pressure less than 60 mm Hg (Fig. 6.2). Five-sixths of the removed blood volume was replaced at a rate of 2 ml/min/kg within forty-five seconds of the hemorrhage. Infusion of hemoglobin-Ringer's (3.7 g/dl oxyhemoglobin) resulted in an immediate rise in blood pressure but was followed by a gradual fall associated

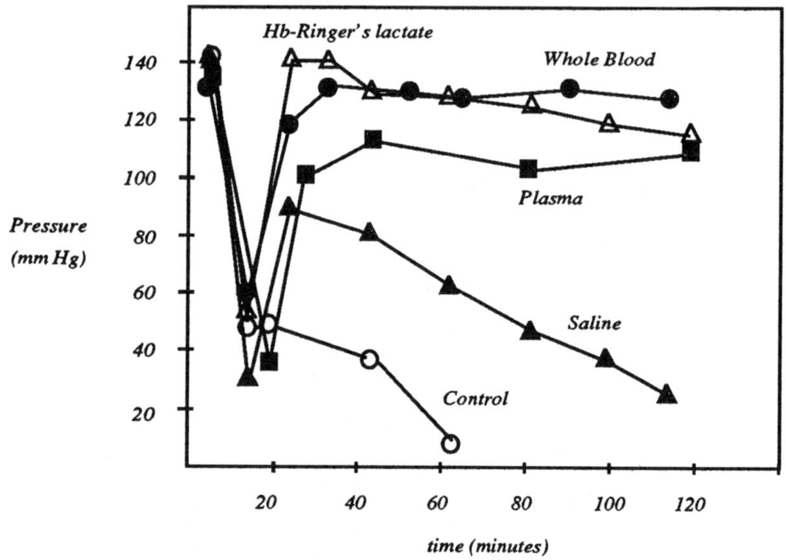

Figure 6.2. Resuscitation of anesthetized cats with whole blood, Hb-Ringer's lactate, plasma, saline, or nothing (*control*). Hb-Ringer's lactate is as effective as whole blood. *Source:* adapted from Buttle et al. (1940).

with respiratory instability. The authors concluded that the results were better than those with normal saline or gum-saline but that the hemoglobin was lost rapidly from the kidneys with both loss of oxygen capacity and renal toxicity. Buttle and his coworkers reached several conclusions that are as important today as they were in 1940: (1) the design of the animal model is important in terms of the rate and site of hemorrhage, length of time the shock state is maintained, and the rate of resuscitation; and (2) renal toxicity clouded any ultimate assessment of the product because long-term recovery was tied more to toxicity than efficacy.

These early studies showed enough promise of efficacy to stimulate workers in the field to continue toward the goal of a red cell substitute. However, before the development of modern purification methods and the methods to modify hemoglobin oxygen affinity and vascular retention serious efficacy studies could not be done.

In 1949 Amberson reviewed his work on hemoglobin solutions (Amberson, Jennings, and Rhode 1949). The product had evolved to one based on human hemoglobin that could be lyophilized (Amberson et al. 1942). The results of hemoglobin injections into fourteen patients were reported in the 1949 paper. Seven received multiple injections, and seven had only one. Among the patients who received multiple injections, five had secondary anemia after hemorrhage. Of these five patients, three showed accelerated erythropoiesis and increased hemoglobin concentration and hematocrit after therapy. In a fourth, bleeding continued, and the erythropoietic response could not be evaluated. Amberson was optimistic about the eventual use of hemoglobin solutions as erythropoietic stimulants.

Perhaps the most interesting patient treated by Amberson was a woman with postpartum hemorrhage in whom 2,300 ml of hemoglobin-saline was given in five injections (Fig. 6.3). Her blood pressure had returned to normal, and she appeared to be recovering when she developed oliguria and uremia and died. Amberson considered this to be the most instructive of his cases because it illustrated both the benefits possible with hemoglobin solutions and also the dangers of intravenous administration.

When better-characterized solutions became available after Rabiner's demonstration of the toxicity of stroma (Rabiner et al. 1967) efficacy demonstrations were repeated (Palani et al. 1974; DeVenuto et al. 1977; DeVenuto, Friedman, and Mellick 1980). Again, these studies showed that animals *could* be kept alive after total exchange of red cells with hemoglobin solutions. In recent years, the focus of experimental questions has sharpened, and the quality of the solutions has improved.

6.2 *Can* It Work? Oxygen Transport

The basic question, *Can hemoglobin solutions work?* can be best examined in the simplest biologic systems such as the ex vivo isolated, perfused heart. Hemoglobin solutions can transport oxygen in such systems (Biro, Beresford-Kroeger, and Smith 1978; Biro and Beresford-Kroeger 1980). For example, Macdonald et al. (1989) used the isolated, perfused rabbit heart for a series of controlled demonstrations of this fact (Fig. 6.4). These investigators perfused the coronary arteries with various test solutions and measured the left ventricular developed pressure as an index of the adequacy of oxygen delivery. Figure 6.4 shows that as the oxygen tension of the perfusing solution is decreased there is a steady loss of

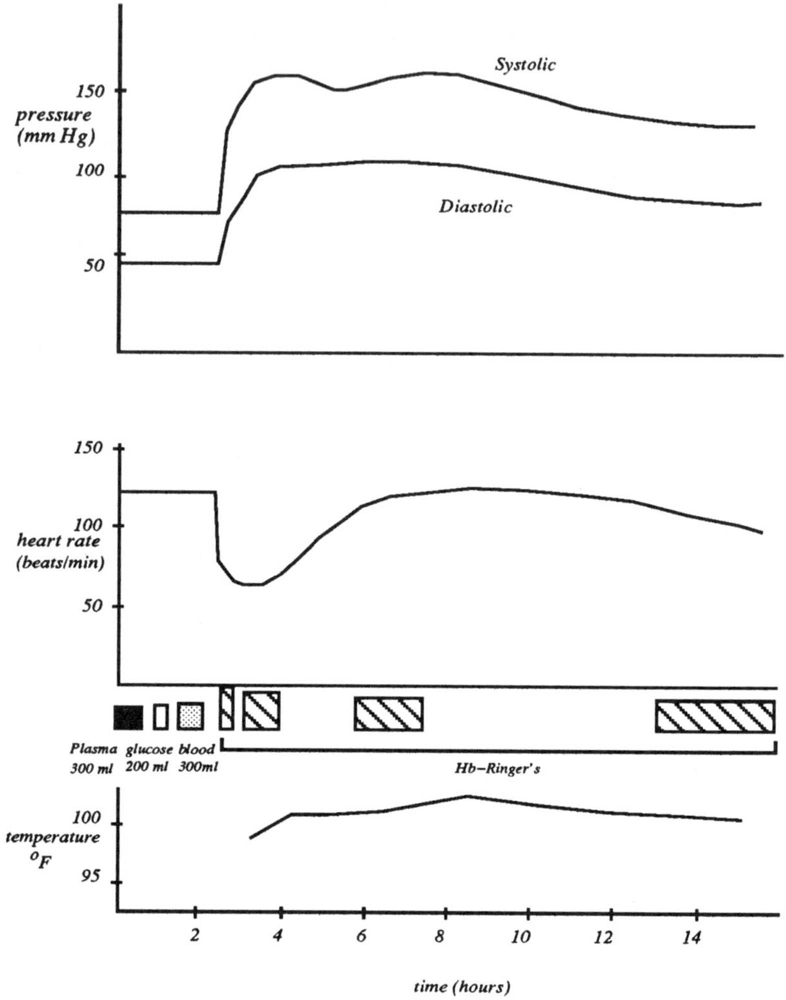

Figure 6.3. Administration of hemoglobin-Ringer's solution to a patient with post-partum hemorrhagic shock. The hemoglobin (*cross-hatched boxes*) was immediately effective in lowering the heart rate and raising the blood pressure whereas glucose, plasma and blood had little effect. *Source*: adapted from Amberson, Jennings, and Rhode (1949).

ventricular function, down to an oxygen tension in the perfusing solution of about 40–50 torr.

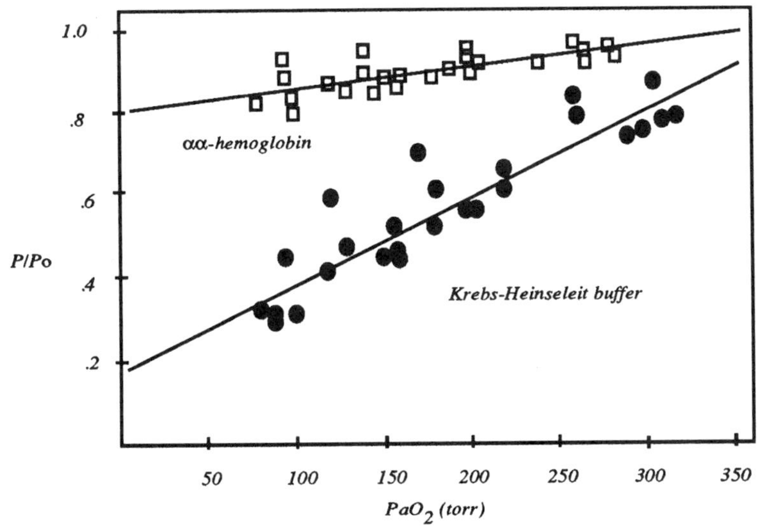

Figure 6.4. Ventricular function (left ventricular developed pressure/control value) with progressive deoxygenation of the perfusing solution in an isolated rabbit heart. Modified hemoglobin delivers more oxygen to the myocardium than buffer alone. Hemoglobin concentration, 1.5 g/dl. *Source:* Macdonald et al. (1989).

Figure 6.4 also shows the same experiment using hemoglobin cross-linked with bis-(3,5-dibromosalicyl)fumarate (DBBF) (see Chapter 5). These data are of interest because the molecular mass (and therefore COP) of the cross-linked hemoglobin is the same as that of the unmodified hemoglobin, but its P_{50} is higher (about 28 torr) compared to hemoglobin A_0 (about 15 torr). Therefore, the data indicate that tissue oxygenation, as measured by left ventricular work, is maintained by the hemoglobin solution, regardless of its oxygen affinity. However, higher mixed venous oxygen tension in the hearts perfused with cross-linked hemoglobin (Table 6.2) shows that tissue oxygenation is better with this solution.

Finally, Macdonald and co-workers (1989) controlled for the presence of protein in the perfusate by perfusing with albumin at the same concentration as the hemoglobin solutions, proving that it is the oxygen-carrying property of hemoglobin which allows myocardial function to be maintained at very low oxygen tensions.

Table 6.2. Oxygen Uptake and Extraction in Isolated Rabbit Hearts Perfused with Modified and Unmodified Hemoglobin Solutions

Solution	PaO_2 (torr)	O_2 Uptake (μm/minute/g)	Extraction Ratio
αα-hemoglobin	559 ± 32	33 ± 5	0.27 ± 0.03
	141 ± 13[a]	32 ± 13	0.42 ± 0.16[b]
Hb A_o	552 ± 37	39 ± 13	0.30 ± 0.09
	141 ± 12[a]	325 ± 2[c]	0.29 ± 0.01

Source: Macdonald (1991).

[a] $p<0.001$
[b] $p=0.016$
[c] $p=0.012$

These studies and many others in the literature demonstrate clearly that hemoglobin-containing solutions *do* transport oxygen to tissues: the answer to the question, *Is it good to perfuse organs with oxygen-carrying solutions?* must be clearly *yes*. However, this is not the question asked by the clinician faced with a patient in shock who has chronic anemia, or who is a candidate for hemodilution during elective surgery. His question is, *Should I administer hemoglobin solution in preference to conventional therapy?* Experiments in isolated, perfused organs will never answer such questions; they will only establish the fact that they *can* be used, not that they *should* be.

6.3 Clinical Applications

6.3.1 Resuscitation

Elia et al. (1974) compared unmodified hemoglobin solution with standard therapy (Ringer's lactate and whole blood) in resuscitating dogs after a severe hemorrhage. The animals were bled to a mean arterial blood pressure of 30 mm Hg and held at that value for 1.5 hours before resuscitation. They found no acid-base or coagulation problems in the hemoglobin group, and the rate and completeness of recovery in these animals were superior to those receiving standard therapy. Hauser and Shomaker (1982) extended these studies with detailed hemodynamic measurements in dogs after rapid hemorrhage (Fig. 6.5). They were able to show that hemoglobin solution was superior to human plasma, whole blood, and Ringer's lactate in restoring blood pressure. These authors concluded that two properties of hemoglobin, COP and oxygen-carrying

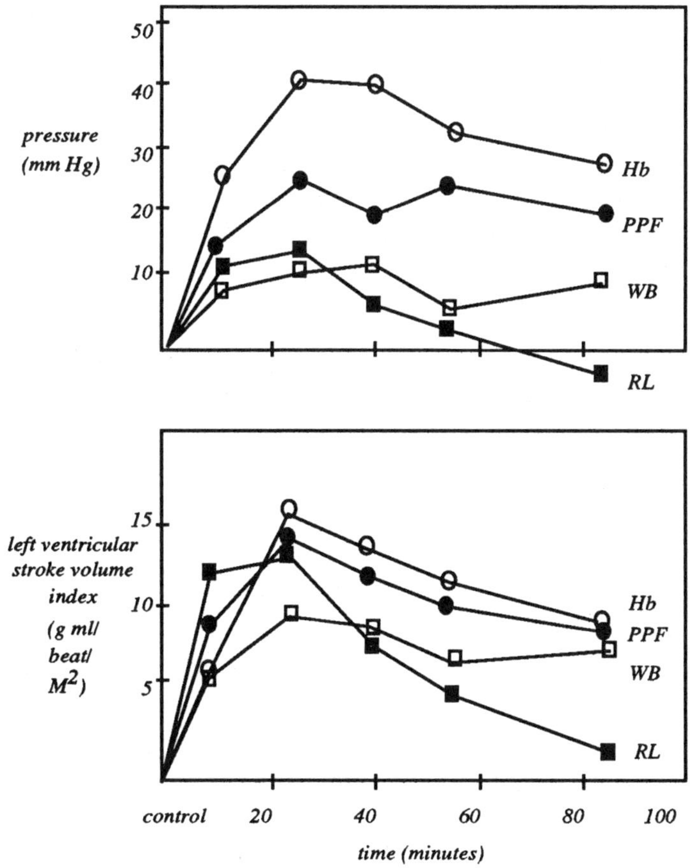

Figure 6.5. Changes in mean arterial blood pressure (*top*) and left ventricular stroke work index (*bottom*) after resuscitation of acutely hypovolemic dogs with hemoglobin (*Hb*), plasma protein fraction (*PPF*), whole blood (*WB*), or Ringer's lactate (*RL*). *Source*: adapted from Hauser and Shoemaker (1982).

capacity, may make it a "nearly ideal" solution for short-term restoration of circulatory oxygen transport. However, 40 percent of the dogs that were successfully resuscitated ultimately died. The authors argued that to be successful solutions should be modified to reduce oxygen affinity, and to prolong vascular persistence.

Later, Odling-Smee and McLarnon (1984) carried out similar studies in dogs but compared the efficacy of dextran 70 with hemoglobin that had been pyridoxylated. They found essentially no difference in the two solutions in their ability to resuscitate the animals, but those animals that received hemoglobin solution had significantly higher mixed venous oxygen tension values after resuscitation. This implies superior oxygen supply to tissues in the hemoglobin-resuscitated animals and agrees with Macdonald's data cited above.

Keipert and Chang (1985) reported a set of measurements of mean arterial pressure during controlled hemorrhage and subsequent resuscitation in conscious rats (Fig. 6.6). About two-thirds of the estimated blood

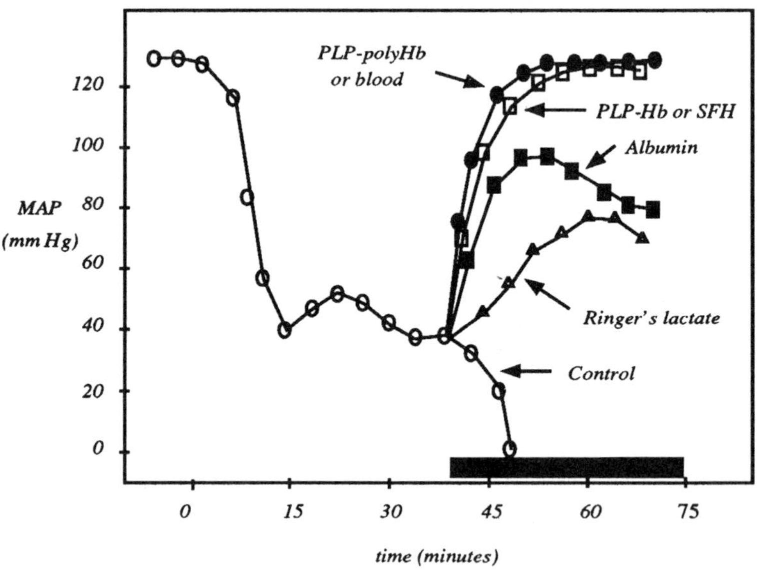

Figure 6.6. Mean arterial blood pressure (*MAP*) in conscious rats. Lethal hemorrhagic shock was induced by removal of two-thirds of the blood volume. After stabilization, animals were resuscitated with the solutions indicated, administered during the time indicated by the *solid bar*. *Source:* Keipert and Chang (1985), with permission.

volume was removed from indwelling femoral artery catheters over a period of about fifteen minutes. After maintenance of the hypotensive state for an additional fifteen minutes, test solutions, in volumes equal to those removed, were reinfused to resuscitate the animals. As Figure 6.6 shows, no therapy was uniformly fatal in these animals. Whole blood and pyridoxylated, polymerized hemoglobin (PLP-polyHb) were equally effective, whereas both albumin and Ringer's lactate were less so. These observations establish that over the short term, the modified hemoglobin solution is as effective as blood and is superior to either pure crystalloid or non-oxygen-carrying colloid.

The simple rat model of acute hemorrhagic shock certainly suggest the efficacy of hemoglobin solutions but raises several other questions. *What if the rate of bleeding were slower (or faster)? What if the the shock state is prolonged?* Most importantly, *What if the degree of hemorrhage is not lethal? Is it still useful to administer hemoglobin solution in preference to crystalloid or other colloid solutions?*

In a variation on this basic model, Marks et al. (1987) studied hemorrhage and resuscitation in dogs. Although they also bled their animals to a mean arterial pressure of 40 mm Hg, this was not lethal. They resuscitated after thirty minutes with whole blood, Ringer's lactate, or pyr-polyHb. Finally, after resuscitation, all animals were given Ringer's lactate to bring the resuscitation volume up to three times that of shed blood. No animals died as a result of the hemorrhage or resuscitation. The authors believed this protocol to be much more realistic than the type of study reported by Keipert and Chang, and they questioned whether hemoglobin solutions could be proved efficacious in ordinary clinical settings.

Some of the adverse effects of hemoglobin solutions could be caused by contaminants. Therefore, Labrude et al. (1988) studied the effect of extensive purification on the outcome of resuscitation in acute hemorrhagic shock. They studied hemoglobin prepared from outdated human blood, the same hemoglobin after coupling with pyridoxal 5'-phosphate (PLP-Hb), and then the coupled material further conjugated to polyethylene glycol (PLP-PEG-Hb). The effect of chromatographic purification of each of the three solutions was also studied. The PLP-PEG-Hb had a concentration of 7 g/dl, pH 7.75, MetHb 7 percent, P_{50} about 15 torr, and molecular mass of about 90,000 daltons. The results (Table 6.3) demonstrate that purification of the hemoglobin solutions is essential to their successful use. Further, the increased molecular mass of the PEG-coupled material prolongs its intravascular retention and therefore its usefulness as a resuscitation solution. This study underscores the need for a well-characterized and highly purified product. Indeed, it suggests that without rigid quality control, interpretation of biologic evaluations might be impossible.

Table 6.3. Short- and Long-term Survival of Rats After Hemorrhagic Shock

Hemorrhage:	60% Blood Volume			80% Blood Volume		
		Survival (minutes ± S.E.[a])			Survival (minutes ± S.E.)	
	n	short	long	*n*	short	long
Ringer's lactate	14	54 ± 6	0			
Human serum albumin	8		8	5	26 ± 3	0
Unmodified Hb	7	640 ± 173	1	8	198 ± 15	0
Purified Hb	6		6	5	240 ± 13	0
PLP-Hb	5	1,245	4	5	430 ± 20	1
Purified PLP-Hb	3	1,320 ± 1,540	1			
PLP-PEG-Hb	3	1,917	0	5	997 ± 158	1
Purified PLP-PEG-Hb	5	[30–48 hours]	2			

Source: data from Labrude et al. (1988).
[a] *S.E.*, standard error of the mean

6.3.2 Intracranial Pressure

Most studies of efficacy concern survival, demonstration of extreme hemodilution, or organ performance. Many studies focus on the heart because it is an organ that can be used readily for ex vivo experiments. However, the heart is well known to be extremely efficient at oxygen extraction, and perhaps adverse effects of hypoxia in the brain should receive more attention. The assessment of the adequacy of oxygen transport to the brain is extremely difficult to design and quantitate because the brain's function cannot be measured as easily as that of the heart or other organs.

Some of the difficulties that will be encountered in using colloid solutions are demonstrated by a comparison of hypertonic saline (7 percent NaCl), normal saline (Prough et al. 1986), or dextran 40 (Gunnar et al. 1987). Resuscitation with hypertonic saline from hemorrhagic shock in dogs leads to rapid stabilization of the cardiovascular system, but the intracranial pressure remains very low relative to animals resuscitated with either normal saline or dextran 40. Altered oncotic pressure or ionic strength of the resuscitation solution could therefore hold special hazards for certain patients such as those with dehydration or intracranial mass lesions.

Many other studies have shown that hemoglobin-based blood substitutes are superior to simple volume expansion in the treatment of hemorrhagic shock in experimental animals (Hauser et al. 1982; Hauser and Shoemaker 1982). Nevertheless, the successful blood substitute must demonstrate similar (or improved) efficacy in humans, when compared with standard therapy, in specific clinical settings. Lethal shock may be the most relevant model in this regard, but it will be difficult to design clinical trials of resuscitation from lethal shock in humans because of the ethical and moral considerations in obtaining informed consent from trauma victims or their families. It seems likely that the first blood substitute that is used in clinical medicine will be the one for which human efficacy and safety can be shown clearly using innovative experimental designs.

6.3.3 Hemodilution

Hemodilution is the replacement of all or a portion of the red cell mass with a solution that does not contain red cells. This therapy has been used extensively in animals to demonstrate efficacy of hemoglobin solutions in transporting oxygen, as in the early studies cited in this chapter. The actual clinical application of hemodilution would be carried out with less than total replacement of the red cell mass, which has no clinical parallel.

After Rabiner demonstrated the superiority of purified hemoglobin solutions (Rabiner et al. 1967), hemodilution studies were undertaken. Some of the studies showed short-term success but because of the short intravascular retention, long-term survival was not good (Holdefer and Dowling 1974). DeVenuto, Moores, Zegna, and Zuck (1977) carried out two hemodilution protocols in rats, one nearly complete (91–93 percent replacement) and the other partial (70–76 percent replacement). In the complete hemodilution, all animals given 5 percent albumin were dead within ten minutes of the procedure, whereas animals diluted with unmodified hemoglobin solution were alive and normally active five hours later.

Subsequent studies by DeVenuto (1982a, 1982b, and Devenuto, Busse, and Zegna 1981) showed that PLP-polyHb with a P_{50} of 19–22 torr extended survival indefinitely in this model; the hemoglobin disappeared from the circulation with a half-time of twenty-five hours. Vogel et al. (1986) also reported that three of four dogs survived indefinitely after total exchange transfusion with PLP-polyHb. Their animals showed unchanged cardiac output, mean arterial pressure and heart rate and a plasma disappearance of hemoglobin of thirty-six hours.

An automated procedure for performance of such hemodilution studies was described by Keipert and Chang (1987). Their procedure employs femoral arterial and venous catheters in the awake rat. Blood is pumped out from the arterial catheter, and test solution is pumped in by the venous catheter such that the near-zero hematocrit state can be reached in approximately ninety minutes. Using this technique, they were able to demonstrate that PLP-polyHb resulted in superior long-term survival after complete hemodilution as compared with albumin, Ringer's lactate, unmodified hemoglobin, or PLP-Hb (see Table 6.4).

Table 6.4. Long-term Survival (as Percent Remaining 8 Days After Various Degrees of Hemodilution in the Conscious Rat)

	Percent hemodilution				
Material	30	40–50	70	80–90	97–100
Albumin	100	60	33	0	0
Ringer's	83	29	0	0	
Hemoglobin[a]	88	40	20		0
PLP-Hb[b]	100	55	22		0
PLP-polyHb[c]	100	80	80	63	50

Source: data from Keipert and Chang (1987), with permission.
[a] Unmodified human hemoglobin solution.
[b] Pyridoxylated human hemoglobin.
[c] Pyridoxylated, polymerized human hemoglobin.

Moores et al. (1982) studied hemodilution of the pig with an unmodified hemoglobin solution. Animals in their study were prepared by bypassing the right ventricle so that oxygenation could be controlled. Even though the hemoglobin solution had a P_{50} of only 14 torr they were able to show that animals hemodiluted about 20 percent (to 5 percent hematocrit) with hemoglobin showed less drop in stroke volume, had much less lactic acid production, and maintained myocardial oxygen uptake better than animals hemodiluted to the same degree with albumin.

Jesch et al. (1982) illustrated both the effectiveness of hemodilution and the importance of lowering affinity. They hemodiluted dogs by removing two-thirds of the blood volume and replacing it with either PLP-polyHb (P_{50} 34.6 torr, COP 54.1 torr) or unmodified hemoglobin (P_{50} 16.9 torr, COP 44.2 torr). Measurements of oxygen tension in skeletal muscle were made using a multiwire platinum electrode. In both groups, the hematocrit fell to about 12 percent and cardiac output and mean arterial pressure were constant. The muscle oxygen tension measurements (Fig. 6.7) showed clearly the superiority of the solution with high P_{50} in maintaining tissue oxygen tension. Long-term survival in the PLP-Hb (five out of six) was also better than in the hemoglobin group (three out of six).

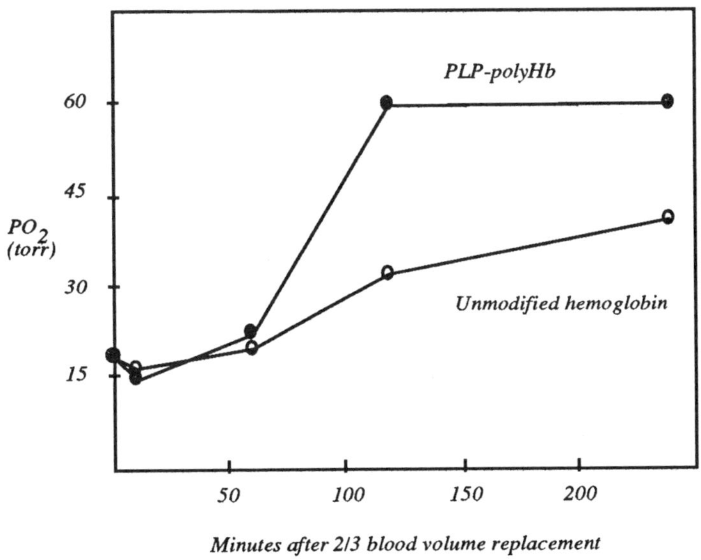

Figure 6.7. Skeletal muscle PO_2 measured at various times after withdrawal of two-thirds of the estimated blood volume and replacement with equal amounts of hemoglobin or PLP-polyHb in the dog. The reduced O_2 affinity of the modified hemoglobin is reflected by a higher tissue PO_2. *Source:* data from Jesch et al. (1982).

Hemodilution experiments similar to those cited in detail above have been carried out by other investigators using different hemoglobin solutions and animal models. Tam, Blumenstein, and Wong (1978), for example, completely exchange-transfused three dogs with a dextran-hemoglobin complex and showed that long-term survival was better than in those exchanged with dextran alone. They also emphasized the vigorous erythropoiesis that followed the procedure, presumably due to the ready availability of iron. Hess and co-workers (1989), using an automated plasma exchange system, showed similar results in pigs completely exchange-transfused with αα–Hb. Sehgal et al. (1986) performed complete exchanges in seven baboons using PLP–polyHb (Table 6.5) and showed preservation of oxygen consumption, blood pressure, and cardiac output. They also calculated that at hematocrits of 10 and 20 percent, their hemoglobin solution accounted for 37–59 and 18–37 percent of the oxygen delivered, respectively.

Table 6.5. Oxygen Transport in Seven Baboons Before and After Exchange-Transfusion with PLP-polyHb.

	Before	After
O_2 consumption (ml/minute)	60.1 ± 8.5	58.0 ± 4.8
MAP (mm Hg)[a]	138 ± 8	140 ± 8
Heart rate (beats/minute)	114 ± 3	117 ± 10
Cardiac output (liters/minute)	1.63 ± 0.3	1.30 ± 0.2

Source: data from Sehgal et al. (1986).
[a] MAP, mean arterial pressure.

6.3.4 Organ Preservation

Hemoglobin solutions may serve well as perfusates for isolated organs for both transplantation applications and in the experimental laboratory. Starnes and co-workers (Tewari et al. 1990; Starnes et al. 1991) compared the efficacy of αα-Hb with red cell suspensions and Krebs-Ringer bicarbonate buffer in maintaining the metabolic integrity of isolated, perfused rat livers (Table 6.6). They found that concentrations of glucose, lactic acid, amino acids, and potassium in the effluent perfusate were the same for livers perfused with red cells (hematocrit 19 percent) and αα-Hb (Hb concentration 7 g/dl). Furthermore, both αα-Hb and red blood cells maintained comparable gas exchange. In contrast, buffer-perfused livers showed reduced oxygen uptake and bile production, reduced glucose utilization, and greater lactic acid production. In addition, morphologic studies showed extensive pathologic changes in the buffer-perfused livers but not in those perfused with αα-Hb or red cells. These authors concluded that hemoglobin solutions were as effective as red blood cells in maintaining the metabolic activity of the ex vivo rat liver. As such, the risk of viral contamination could be eliminated using these solutions. Hemoglobin solutions have also been shown to be useful in the preservation of canine hearts (Holdefer and Dowling 1974).

Table 6.6. Perfusion of the Isolated Rat Liver With Red Blood Cells (RBC), αα-Hb Solution, and Krebs-Ringer Bicarbonate (KRB) Buffer

Perfusate (*n*)	Glucose Outflow (nmol/g)	Lactate Production (nmol/g)	K^+ Outflow (μmol/g)	O_2 Uptake (μl/minute)
RBC	49.4 ± 26.4	3.2 ± 17.4	40.4 ± 13.1	52.5 ± 5.3
αα–Hb	61.7 ± 44.6	35.7 ± 14.1	76.0 ± 8.6	58.3 ± 3.9
KRB	222.4 ± 59.3	124.6 ± 40.8	158.0 ± 29.0	16.6 ± 1.3

Source: data from Tewari et al. (1990).

6.4 Are Hemoglobin-based Red Cell Substitutes Better Than Other Therapy?

Studies comparing different resuscitation solutions have been difficult to perform and interpret for at least two reasons. First, hemoglobin solutions whose quality was sufficiently high that results were not marred by toxicity have been available only recently. Second, models of efficacy often use survival as the end point; survival can discriminate only when the protocol involves biologic stress not commonly encountered clinically. For example, Gerald Moss et al. (1976) showed that baboons could survive hemodilution with albumin solution to a hematocrit of 6 percent, and further hemodilution is required in order to show the advantages of hemoglobin solution in survival rates.

One comparative study was reported recently (Watzek and Steinbereithner 1988) in which the ability of PLP-Hb (Biotest), Fluosol-DA 20%, and dextran 60 were studied with regard to their ability to resuscitate rabbits after the induction of hemorrhagic shock. Each group of animals received either isovolemic or hypervolemic fluid administration (Table 6.7). The authors concluded that in order to be effective, PLP-polyHb and Fluosol-DA 20% needed to be given in hypervolemic quantities, but had no appreciable advantage over dextran.

Table 6.7. Survival of Rabbits (in Minutes) after Resuscitation from Hemorrhagic Shock with Various Solutions

Treatment	Isovolemic		Hypervolemic	
	n	minutes	*n*	minutes
None	10	168	10	172
Dextran 60	10	914	10	712
Fluosol-DA 20%	10	415	10	909
PLP-polyHb	10	377	10	1,056

Source: data from Watzek and Steinbereithner (1988).

George Biro (1982) compared 8 percent hemoglobin, Fluosol-DA 20% and dextran 70 in their ability to transport oxygen to the hearts of anesthetized dogs. Hemodilution and viscosity were similar for all three solutions, but only the dextran 70 and Fluosol-DA 20%-diluted dogs showed an increase in cardiac output. As a result, the hemoglobin-diluted dogs showed inadequate oxygen supply, suggested by a fall in coronary oxygen tension. In this study, as with similar ones, the hemoglobin solution was prepared according to Rabiner et al. (1967) and therefore, as later studies show, had high oxygen affinity.

A reperfusion experiment by the same group (Biro and Beresford-Kroeger 1980) came to different conclusions. In this study, the left anterior descending coronary artery of anesthetized dogs was occluded for one hour, and then a rapid exchange transfusion with hemoglobin, dextran 70, or whole blood was carried out. After the procedure, blood flow to the ischemic zone, measured by the microsphere technique, increased in the hemoglobin and dextran 70 animals but not in those reperfused with whole blood. The greatest improvement was seen in the hemoglobin group: endocardial flow increased by 83 percent and epicardial flow by 45 percent. The hemoglobin animals also showed the least increase in creatine phosphokinase and a return to preocclusion left ventricular function. The authors believed that the acute reduction in viscosity was probably important in the hemoglobin group. Similar data were reported by Feola, Azarr, and Wiener (1979), who also showed an increased myocardial oxygen tension and a reduction in the presumptive infarct volume in hemoglobin-treated hearts compared with those perfused with dextran 70 or whole blood.

Greenburg et al. (1978) compared the ability of pyridoxylated hemoglobin with Ringer's lactate (twice volume) and whole blood in resuscitation of dogs after induction of acute hemorrhagic shock (blood pressure less than 50 mm Hg for ninety minutes). They found no differences as defined by hemodynamics (blood pressure, heart rate, central venous pressure), oxygen delivery (P_{50}, hemoglobin, hematocrit), and blood gases over a period of ninety minutes after resuscitation. These authors attributed the success to the near-physiologic P_{50} (31.2 torr) and prolonged vascular retention (half-life of 140 minutes). They concluded that since hemoglobin is the only solution capable of sustaining life at zero hematocrit, the data support the claim that pyridoxylated hemoglobin was ready for clinical evaluation.

Chapter 7

The Metabolism of Hemoglobin

In 1870, the great French physiologist Paul Bert asserted that circulating hemoglobin, freed from the red cell, is toxic (Bert 1879). He came to this conclusion after a series of experiments in which dogs were hemorrhaged until very near death and then revived with either hemolyzed blood or serum. He claimed that the serum was more effective, but the data were not quantitative. Subsequent experiments by Barratt (Barratt and Yorke 1909) and Roger (1919) supported Bert's views but used rabbits, animals shown later to be unusually sensitive to hemolysed blood. The mechanism of toxicity of hemolysed blood subsequently received considerable attention because of the frequency of hemolytic transfusion reactions.

As early as 1916 Sellards noted that "the most striking feature about the literature is the frequency of contradictions in the results obtained by various investigators. Some investigators maintain that hemoglobin is distinctly toxic, and that animals can easily be killed with solutions of their own hemoglobin" (Sellards and Minot 1916). Yet Sellards and others showed that many hemoglobin infusions were well tolerated. Recently, a number of investigators have suggested that heme, whether protein-bound or free, could promote the formation of toxic oxygen radicals, limiting the promise of cell-free hemoglobin as a blood substitute (Faasen et al. 1988). Thus, the question of whether hemoglobin itself is toxic is critical.

Hemoglobin solutions in rabbits have been reported to cause problems, ranging from a pyrogen (febrile) response to sudden death. Extravasation in many tissues, including skin, eye, and other organs, has been reported. Renal failure, particularly after the infusion of "stroma-free" hemoglobin, is predictable, possibly because of the presence of residual stromal materials (Feola, Simoni, Canizaro, et al. 1988; Feola, Simoni, Tran, et al. 1988). Hepatic necrosis has been observed by almost all workers in the field, but some believe that the typical lesion (centrolobular necrosis) is transient and reversible.

Normally, red cells are removed from the body by the reticuloendothelial system. In humans, the main sites of reticuloendothelial activity are the spleen, liver, bone marrow, and kidney (Fig. 7.1). Senescent red blood cells are destroyed, iron is recycled for use, and globin is digested by proteolytic enzymes. In the liver cell, the protoporphyrin of heme is cleaved to produce biliverdin, an open-chain tetrapyrrole compound, which is promptly converted to bilirubin and excreted in the feces as urobilinogen (Fig. 7.2). This process generates carbon monoxide, which is transported as carboxyhemoglobin to the lung, in which it is exchanged for oxygen.

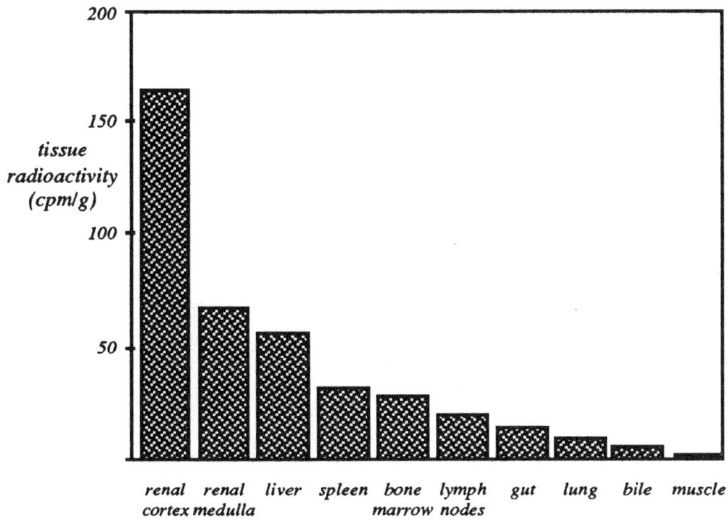

Figure 7.1. Organ distribution of unmodified hemoglobin. Dog hemoglobin was labeled with ^{51}Cr, purified and reinfused. Animals were killed after twenty-four hours to quantitate tissue hemoglobin content. *Source*: data from Anderson, Mouritzen, and Gabrielli (1966).

In hemolytic states, hemoglobin is free in the plasma, and clearance is by different mechanisms (Crosby and Dameshek 1951). If hemoglobin-based red cell substitutes are developed successfully, massive infusions of protein will be needed, particularly for resuscitation from hemorrhage. How this protein will be metabolized and cleared is not necessarily an extrapolation of known mechanisms. Remarkably, few data exist in the literature to follow the metabolic fate of large hemoglobin infusions.

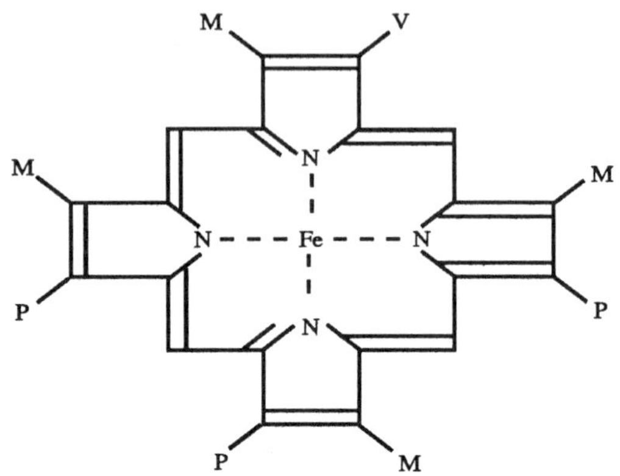

Heme

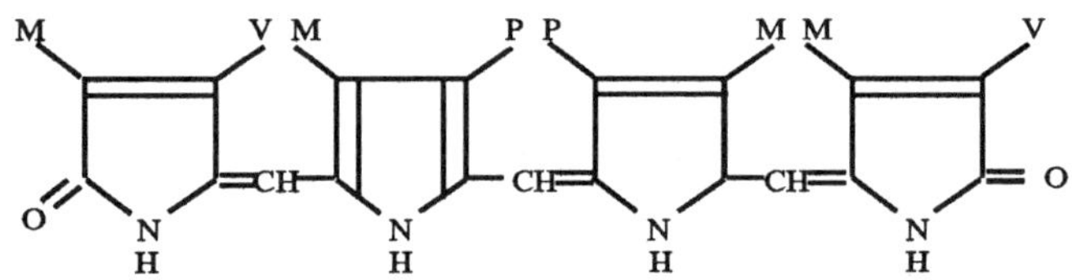

Biliverdin IXα

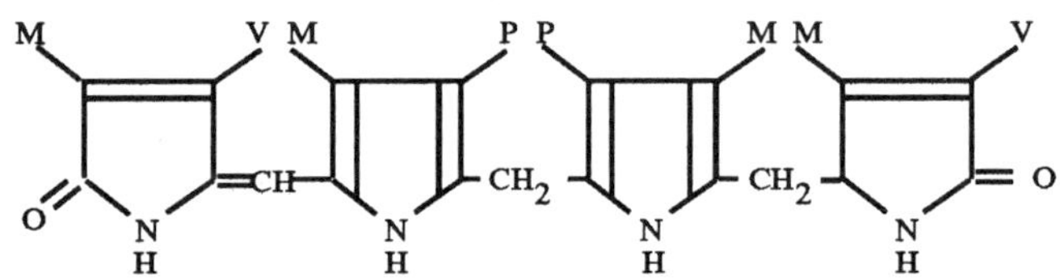

Bilirubin IXα

Figure 7.2. Breakdown of heme. Heme is degraded first to biliverdin IXα and then to the final degradation product, bilirubin IXα. *M*, methyl; *P*, propionic acid; *V*, vinyl.

7.1 Histology

When hemoglobin is injected into intact animals, it is distributed widely in tissues (Fig. 7.1). Although hemoglobin can be found in virtually all tissues, only liver and kidney seem to show evidence of cell damage. Friedman et al. (1977) found dense osmiophilic granules in the proximal tubular cells of rat kidneys one hour after a 75 percent exchange transfusion with "crystalline" hemoglobin (DeVenuto, Moores, Zegna, and Zuck 1977). These were still present in twenty-four hours. Tubular obstruction also occurs immediately, as hemoglobin is cleared by the kidney. In the liver, centrolobular necrosis occurs as hemoglobin is cleared, and Friedman and co-workers believed that this was hypoxic damage. They found no histologic alterations in the hippocampus, cerebellum, or cerebral cortex.

7.2 Plasma Transport of Heme and Hemoglobin

In humans, free hemoglobin and heme do not circulate. Heme may be released from hemoglobin under some circumstances, but its solubility in aqueous solution is very low. Therefore, it is usually not present unbound even during brisk intravascular hemolysis.

Mechanisms exist to remove free hemoglobin and heme from the circulation to prevent potential oxidative damage to tissues. These mechanisms normally handle very small amounts. Much of what is known about the clearance of hemoglobin and heme in humans is derived from studies on intravascular red cell hemolysis. In the case of large volume replacement, enormous amounts of chemically modified hemoglobin would be presented for clearance. How these large volumes would be handled is not clear.

Plasma hemoglobin is normally removed by several mechanisms (Fig. 7.3). $\alpha_2\beta_2$ molecules dissociate into $\alpha\beta$ dimers that can be bound by the serum protein, haptoglobin. When haptoglobin is saturated, $\alpha\beta$ dimers may be filtered in the glomerulus and then reabsorbed by cells of the proximal tubule. When the reabsorptive capacity is exceeded, hemoglobin appears in the urine. Heme iron of $\alpha\beta$ dimers in the plasma is oxidized to Fe^{3+} and the heme is transferred to albumin to form methemalbumin, and to hemopexin. Hemopexin carries Fe^{3+} to tissue sites of metabolism for subsequent use in the synthesis of heme proteins. Some of the Fe^{3+} may be released from heme and bound to transferrin. Thus, a number of breakdown products or complexes must be either metabolized or eliminated. These are listed in Table 7.1.

7.2.1 $\alpha\beta$-Haptoglobin Complex

$\alpha\beta$ dimers are bound readily to haptoglobin. The complexes are taken up by the reticuloendothelial cells, mainly in the liver but also in the bone marrow and spleen. Inside the cells, heme reaches the microsomes, in which its conversion to bilirubin is initiated by the enzyme heme oxygenase. Goldberg, Dunning and Bunn 1988) proposed that heme oxygenase is the "trigger" for erythropoietin synthesis and that it could explain why free hemoglobin or methemoglobin appears to stimulate erythropoiesis (Gould, Sehgal et al. 1986).

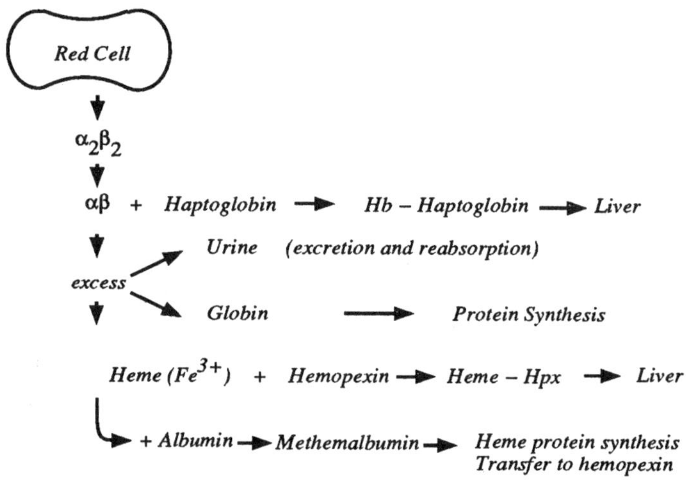

Figure 7.3. Normal removal of hemoglobin from the circulation. In low concentration, $\alpha_2\beta_2$ tetramers dissociate to $\alpha\beta$ dimers, which are bound to haptoglobin and are cleared mainly by the kidney but also by other tissues. When the haptoglobin mechanism is saturated, excess $\alpha\beta$ dimers are filtered in the kidney, some are taken up by the tubule cells, and others appear in the urine. Heme that dissociates from hemoglobin is bound to hemopexin and albumin, transported to the liver, and degraded further there.

7.2.2 Heme-binding Proteins

Albumin is a single-chain protein, molecular mass of 68,000 daltons, composed of 585 amino acids with seventeen disulfide bridges. Its normal concentration in the plasma is about 4 g/dl. Albumin can bind free heme and bilirubin at a high affinity site (dissociation constant 10^{-2} μM/liter; Adams and Berman 1980) between amino acid residues 198 and 308, but there may be other sites with lower affinity (Beaven et al. 1974). The gene that controls its synthesis is located on human chromosome 4.

Table 7.1. Hemoglobin Components That Are Cleared from the Plasma

αβ Dimers
αβ-Haptoglobin complex
Heme-albumin complex
Heme-hemopexin complex
Free heme
Fe^{3+}
Fe^{3+}-transferrin

Hemopexin is a single-chain glycoprotein with a molecular mass of 60,000 daltons, containing about 20 percent carbohydrate (sialic acid, mannose, galactose, fructose, and hexosamine). It is present in the plasma at a concentration of about 4–15 g/dl. The heme binding site is probably near the amino-terminus. It shows very weak peroxidase activity and no catalase activity. Its synthesis is controlled by a single gene on human chromosome 11 (Altruda et al. 1988). Heme is bound much more tightly to hemopexin (dissociation constant $< 10^{-10}$ μM/liter (Hrkal, Vodrazka, and Kalousek 1974) than it is to albumin.

Heme groups in methemoglobin may dissociate from the globin and become bound to hemopexin and albumin. Globin has a high affinity for heme-Fe^{3+} (dissociation constant 10^{-13} M/liter (Hrkal, Vodrazka, and Kalousek 1974). β globin loses heme-Fe^{3+} faster than α globin (Bunn and Jandl 1968), but α globin oxidizes about ten times faster (Mansouri and Winterhalter 1973). Thus, it is likely that heme will not be transferred out of globin unless another protein with a high affinity such as albumin or hemopexin is available. In blood substitute therapy, those proteins might be "swamped out," and heme transfer might not occur. It would be of interest to determine whether tissue cells such as endothelium have high-affinity heme-binding sites.

New studies (Benesch and Kwong 1990) suggest that globin structure in modified and mutant hemoglobins may affect the tightness of the heme-globin linkage. Benesch and Kwong compared methemoglobin A_0, a mutant hemoglobin (Rothschild, β^{37} Trp–Arg), and hemoglobins cross-linked with two reagents, 2-nor-2-formylpyridoxal 5'-phosphate

(NFPLP) and (bis-PL)P_4 (see Chapter 5). They found that both of the cross-linked hemoglobins had increased heme-globin stability, whereas the mutant had decreased stability (Fig. 7.4). It is tempting to speculate that this dissociation might be related to toxicity if heme itself is a major source of toxicity, but additional studies will have to be done to correlate this dissociation with biologic effects.

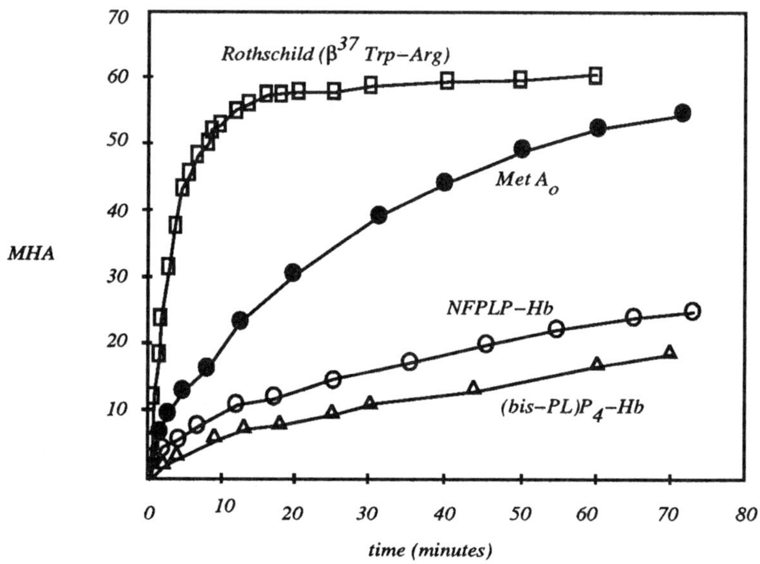

Figure 7.4. Heme exchange rates of different hemoglobins with human serum albumin, measured as percent methemalbumin (*MHA*). Both modified hemoglobins demonstrate reduced rates of heme loss. Conditions: 0.05 mM methemoglobin and albumin. *Source:* Benesch and Kwong (1990), with permission.

7.3 Renal Handling of Hemoglobin

The capacity of the plasma proteins to bind hemoglobin is about 128 mg/dl (Lathem 1959; Lathem and Worley 1959). When the hemoglobin concentration exceeds that value it is free in the plasma and may be filtered in the kidney as αβ dimers. In humans, the threshold for filtration ranges from 0 to 54 mg/dl of free hemoglobin and averages 27 mg/dl. This is equivalent to a total plasma hemoglobin of about 155 mg/dl. In the plasma it is bound to many proteins, including haptoglobin and albumin.

Homer Smith (1951) raised the question of why hemoglobin appears in the urine at all when albumin, whose molecular weight is about the same, does not. Even in the nephrotic syndrome, in which albumin appears in the urine in large amounts, hemoglobin is not filtered in the glomerulus (Brandt, Frank, and Lichtman 1950). This is because the appearance of proteins in the glomerular filtrate is not a simple filtration; the glomerular capillary wall restricts the passage of polyanions more than that of neutral macromolecules because of their net negative charge. Thus, at a pH of 7.4, about the isoionic point for hemoglobin, albumin has a molecular charge of -19. These two molecules have about the same molecular radius (Deen, Satvat, and Jamieson 1980).

Bunn, Esham, and Bull (1969) extended the understanding of the renal handling of hemoglobin by demonstrating that formation of αβ dimers (molecular weight 32,000) is a necessary requirement for glomerular filtration. They modified labeled human hemoglobin with bis(N-maleimidomethyl)ether, injected it into rats, and followed its course of disappearance (Fig. 7.5). These data were the first to show clearly that

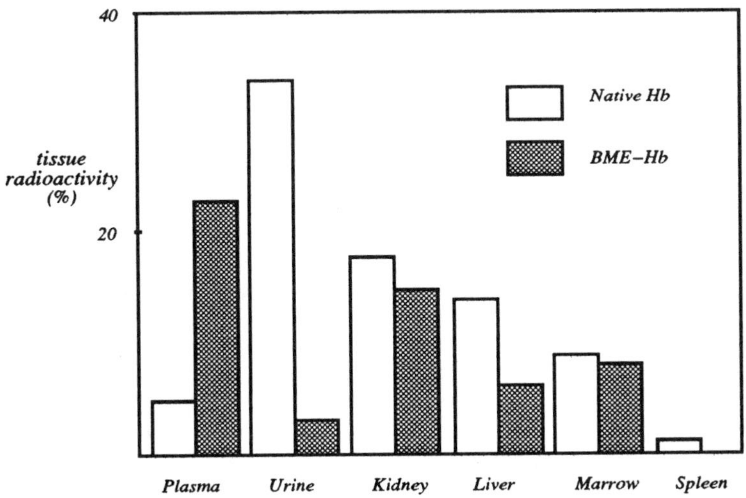

Figure 7.5. Tissue distribution of native hemoglobin and hemoglobin cross-linked with bis(N-maleimidomethyl)ether (BME-Hb) in the rat. Note the differences between the two hemoglobins in regard to prolonged retention in the plasma and reduced clearance in the urine. *Source:* data from Bunn and Jandl (1967).

modification of the hemoglobin molecule to prevent its dissociation into $\alpha\beta$ dimers prolongs its plasma disappearance. Note, however, in Figure 7.5, that an appreciable amount of the modified protein does appear in the kidney even though the clearance in the urine is largely prevented.

Whether or not hemoglobin is reabsorbed in the kidney tubules was debated for some time. Although the reabsorption rate is probably small, some is clearly taken up by tubular cells, as illustrated by microscopic studies (Friedman et al. 1979; 1977; Friedman and DeVenuto 1982), the finding of hemosiderin in tubular cells after severe hemolysis (Goodwin, Alston, and Semens 1950), and by stop-flow experiments (Lathem et al. 1960). This uptake is very important for the proposed mechanism of toxicity involving oxygen free radicals (see below).

After filtration in the glomerulus, $\alpha\beta$ dimers pass down the tubule and, as the pH drops, iron oxidizes giving a positive reaction with Prussian blue (Williams and Kent 1981). Hemoglobin, concentrated in the tubules, is taken up at the brush border of the tubular epithelial cells and transported into vacuoles (Fig. 7.6). These vacuoles enlarge and eventually become "droplets" (Oliver, MacDowell, and Lee 1954) containing degraded hemoglobin, phospholipid, and ferritin (Miller 1960).

7.4 The Metabolic Fate of Modified Hemoglobin

Even though the anticipated use of modified hemoglobin as a plasma expander after hemorrhagic shock or in elective hemodilution would result in administration of massive doses, surprisingly little is known about the metabolic fate of these products. Perhaps the difficulty of preparing labeled hemoglobin is part of the explanation for this lack of information.

To follow the fate of the various components of hemoglobin, Bunn and Jandl (1967) labeled unmodified hemoglobin either with ^{59}Fe (heme), [^{14}C] leucine (globin), or [^{14}C] glycine (porphyrin). When these materials were injected into haptoglobin-depleted rats, they found that nearly half the ^{59}Fe was trapped in the kidneys and that complete disappearance required several weeks ($t_{1/2}$ = 30 days). In contrast, the porphyrin and globin were catabolized more quickly ($t_{1/2}$ = 1 hour). In a similar study, Anderson, Mouritzen, and Gabrielli (1966) reinfused purified, chromium-labeled dog hemoglobin and measured the tissue localization twenty-four hours later (Fig. 7.1). They showed that hemoglobin is deposited widely in many tissues but that the renal cortex contained more than twice the radioactivity of any other organs.

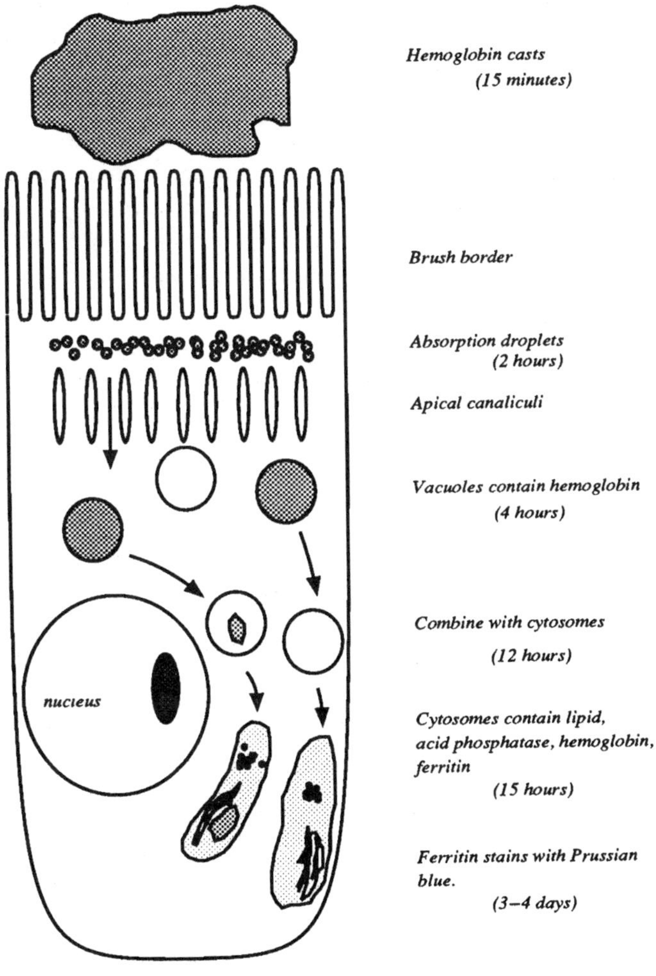

Figure 7.6. Fate of hemoglobin in renal tubular cells. Hemoglobin is reabsorbed across the brush border into cytoplasmic vacuoles that eventually form autosomes. Hemoglobin is degraded within the autosomes.

More recently, Keipert, Verosky, and Triner (1989) compared the organ distribution of pyridoxylated hemoglobin (PLP-Hb) and hemoglobin modified with NFPLP (NFPLP-Hb). These two molecules differ in that the NFPLP-Hb is cross-linked covalently between β chains whereas in the PLP-Hb, the PLP group attaches only to one β chain (see Chapter 5). Keipert and his colleagues found that the plasma retention of NFPLP was three times longer than that of PLP-Hb and that virtually none of the cross-linked material appears in the urine. Its distribution nine hours after injection was mainly in the liver, spleen, and kidneys (Fig. 7.7). Bleeker et al. (1989) also found the prolonged disappearance of NFPLP-Hb but discovered that the accumulation in the kidney was less than that of unmodified hemoglobin and that there was a rapid appearance of NFPLP-Hb in the lymph. More studies of this type are urgently needed to identify which organs are at risk for toxicity from specific hemoglobin products.

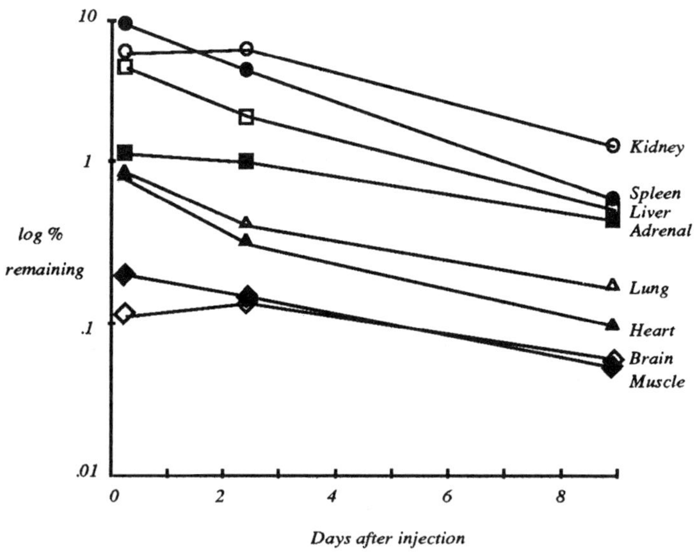

Figure 7.7. Disappearance of ^3H from NFPLP-Hb from various tissues. The label was introduced in the NFPLP cross-link. *Source*: Keipert and Triner (1989), with permission.

7.5 Tissue Metabolism of Heme

Hemopexin and albumin carry heme to the liver, in which it is degraded in hepatocytes. Although albumin-heme may be taken up directly at tissue sites, it is more likely that heme is transferred from albumin to apohemopexin as it is available and then transferred to liver cells.

Heme is taken up by hepatocytes (Fig. 7.8) either bound to hemopexin or albumin or as part of the $\alpha\beta$ dimer-haptoglobin complex (Morgan et al. 1976). The fate of heme-hemopexin complex is not yet entirely clear (Muller-Eberhard and Nikkila 1989). The heme-protein complexes are probably bound to specific cellular receptor sites, internalized briefly, and then give up their heme to intracellular proteins. The plasma proteins can then be "recycled" to bind more heme.

Within the hepatocyte, heme is broken down to bilirubin by a series of enzymatic steps (Fig. 7.2). Bilirubin is secreted into the bile, which appears in the feces. When large doses of free heme are administered, however, undegraded heme may appear in the feces via the bile (McCormack et al. 1982). Inhibitors of heme oxygenase may add further to the liver's inability to degrade heme (Drummond 1989). A necessary step in bilirubin secretion is its conjugation to uridine diphosphate glucuronosyl transferase. In the intestine, the glucuronide is degraded further by bacteria.

7.6 Heme Toxicity

Within tissue cells, heme binds to a number of cytosolic proteins (Muller-Eberhard and Nikkila 1989). Z-protein, also known as fatty acid-binding protein (FABP), is a nonglycosylated, low molecular mass (14,184 daltons) protein that comprises 3 percent of total cytosolic proteins in the liver (Levi, Gatmaitan, and Arias 1969) and other tissues (Bass 1988). Although FABP binds a number of molecules its affinity for heme is particularly high (dissociation constant 10^{-4} μM/liter (Vincent et al. 1988).

Heme seems to be much more toxic than hemoglobin. Early studies (Corcoran and Page 1945) showed that hematin injected into dogs causes dilatation and congestion of small vessels, hemorrhages, and thromboses, and, when taken up by reticuloendothelial cells, it may persist there for prolonged periods of time. Valuable information about the toxicity of heme may be obtained from those porphyria patients who are treated with hemin (Bonkowsky et al. 1971). In these people heme has been shown to cause coagulopathies (Morris, Dudley, and Pearson 1981), disaggregate spectrin (Avissar et al. 1984), activate the factor XII-dependent pathway of coagulation (Becker et al. 1985), aggregate platelets (Neely et al. 1984), and lyse red cells (Chou and Fitch 1981; Fitch et al. 1983). The mechanism of these toxic effects may have in common the formation of activated oxygen species (Halliwell and Gutteridge 1984).

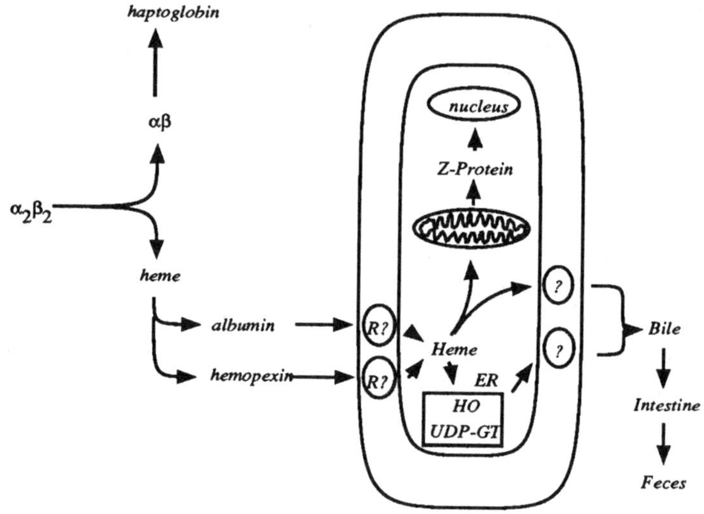

Figure 7.8. Uptake of hemoglobin by the liver cell. Heme is transported to the hepatocyte membrane by hemopexin and albumin. After uptake by the cell, it is either degraded by heme oxygenase *(HO)* in the cytoplasmic reticulum (*ER*), bound to UDP by UDP-glucuronosyl transferase (*UDP-GT*) and excreted into the bile, or it is taken up by the mitochondrion, where it is used in hematoprotein synthesis. Some heme is bound to Z-protein, which may play a role in intranuclear regulation of protein synthesis. *Source:* adapted from Muller-Eberhard and Nikkila (1989).

Apparently it is not necessary for iron to be released from heme to be toxic. Thus, heme is a stronger oxidant than are ferric salts (Beppu, Nagoya, and Kikugawa 1986; Vincent et al. 1988), and heme appears to promote thiobarbituric acid-reacting substances (TBARS) (Vincent et al. 1988). Figure 7.9 shows the catalytic effect of heme in lipid peroxidation (Vincent 1989). At a high concentration of heme, the activity is reduced, consistent with consumption of the oxidizing species of heme itself as well as with further degradation of heme.

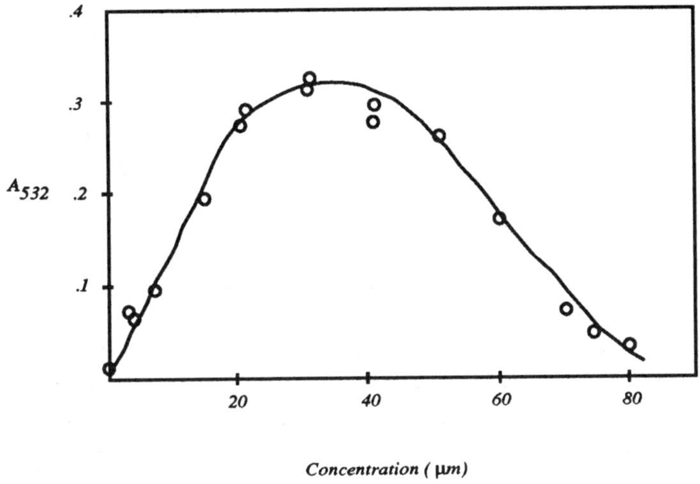

Figure 7.9. Catalytic effect of heme in lipid peroxidation. Rat liver microsomes were incubated with H_2O_2, and lipid peroxidation was measured as TBARS as absorbance at 532 nm. *Source:* adapted from Vincent (1989).

Free heme can also partition into membranes (Rose et al. 1985) and cross-link proteins (Beppu, Nagoya, and Kikugawa 1986; Chui and Lubin 1989). But heme cannot participate in peroxidative catalysis when it is bound to hemopexin or albumin, and it has reduced activity when bound to albumin (Vincent 1989). In sustained hemolysis or possibly after infusion of large quantities of free hemoglobin, the hemopexin concentration falls, and the concentration of free heme may be high (Muller-Eberhard 1970). In these circumstances, heme toxicity could be a real danger.

7.6.1 Activated Oxygen

The reduction of oxygen to hydrogen peroxide is a fundamental process that requires four electrons and releases a large amount of energy (George and Schejter 1964). The reaction can be divided into four sequential steps: formation of (1) superoxide radical, $O_2^{\cdot -}$, (2) peroxide, $O_2^{=}$; (3) hydroxyl radical, $HO^{\cdot}$, and (4) H_2O. Only the first step, superoxide formation, requires energy. Two molecules of superoxide can react to form peroxide and singlet oxygen, another form of activated oxygen:

$$O_2^{\cdot -} + O_2^{\cdot -} \longrightarrow O_2^{=} + O_2 \qquad (1)$$

Superoxide also reacts with peroxide to form $HO^{\cdot}$, the most powerful oxidizing agent in the series. These molecules together are known as activated oxygen. They are interconverted easily, and it is difficult to determine which is responsible for specific biologic effects.

7.6.2 Methemoglobin Formation as a Source of Activated Oxygen

Normally, about 3 percent of the body's hemoglobin is converted to methemoglobin ($Fe^{2+} \longrightarrow Fe^{3+}$) per day (Carrell, Winterbourn, and Rachmilewitz 1975), and this process can be a continual source of $O_2^{\cdot}$. According to this mechanism, an electron in the $Fe\text{-}O_2$ bond is polarized toward the oxygen molecule. This electron is normally returned to the iron when oxygen is released, but occasionally when water or small ions enter the heme pocket for a variety of reasons, the oxygen may leave with the electron as $O_2^{\cdot -}$, and the iron will be in its oxidized Fe^{3+} state (Weiss 1980; Mistra and Fridovich 1972; Wever, Oudega, and VanGelder 1973).

In the red cell this constant supply of $O_2^{\cdot -}$ is reduced by methemoglobin reductase. When hemoglobin is free in the circulation, without its cellular environment the reducing systems are not available, and the production of superoxide can be expected to proceed unabated.

7.6.3 The Role of Heme in Activated Oxygen Formation

Whether or not heme-protein complexes promote lipid peroxidation depends on the affinity of heme binding by the protein (Vincent 1989). Thus, hemopexin has no activity, and the albumin-heme complex enhances peroxidation. Like heme, methemoglobin and myoglobin are ineffective in lipid peroxidation in a high concentration (Kanner and Harel 1985) but reduced hemoglobin has been proposed to be a Fenton reagent (Sadrzadeh et al. 1984). Hemoglobin (but not methemoglobin) promotes $HO^{\cdot}$ formation in the presence of xanthine-xanthine oxidase, and this activity can be prevented by the addition of haptoglobin (haptoglobin binds hemoglobin dimers), carbon monoxide, or catalase (superoxide dismutase had no effect). Thus, heme (Fe^{2+}) probably acts directly on hydrogen peroxide, and Sadrzadeh et al. suggested that haptoglobin might be important in preventing such hemoglobin-mediated oxidation in vivo, for example, in areas of inflammation.

In certain anemias in which hemoglobin is unstable because of structural alterations or because of certain red cell enzyme deficiencies, precipitates form within the cell which reduce its flexibility and lead to eventual premature destruction. These particulates (Heinz bodies) have been studied in detail and found to contain hemichromes, insoluble forms of methemoglobin (Fig. 7.10).

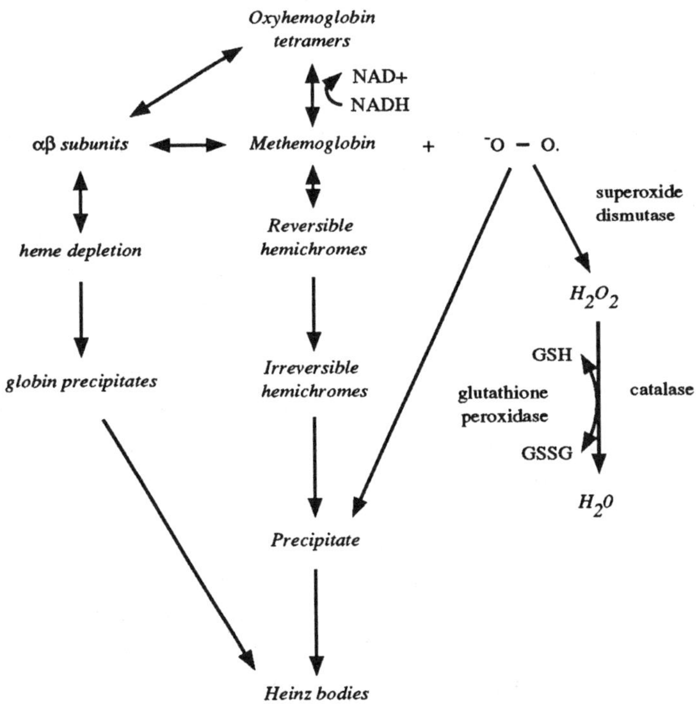

Figure 7.10. Oxidation and degradation of hemoglobin within red cells. In some hemolytic anemias, methemoglobin forms hemichromes which may form insoluble precipitates. Normally, superoxide dismutase, catalase, and glutathione peroxidase (*GSH*) protect against this degradation. In the cell-free condition, this protection would not be available.

Within the sickled red blood cell, hemichromes may contribute to the generation of O_2^-, HO$^\cdot$, and H_2O_2 (Hebbel et al. 1982). Hebbel et al. suggested that the constant cycling of $HbO_2 \leftrightarrow$ MetHb (cyanide ion blocks the effect) is a source of O_2^- (Carrell, Winterbourn, and Rachmilewitz 1975) and that hemichrome (Fe^{3+}) is probably formed at the expense of O_2^- formation (Mistra and Fridovich 1972; Wever, Oudega, and VanGelder 1973; Brunori et al. 1975). Hebbel and colleagues suggested that HO$^\cdot$ might have been generated further from the interaction of Fe^{2+} and hydrogen peroxide (see Chapter 8).

7.7 Red Cell Substitutes

If heme (as hemoglobin) promotes the formation of toxic oxygen radicals, then it would seem inadvisable to infuse it in large quantities as a resuscitation solution in hemorrhagic shock; both iron and oxygen would be made available. In fact, this application is precisely the major goal of many research and development programs today. Hedlund and colleagues (Faasen et al. 1988) were particularly vocal in their warnings on this point.

Indirect evidence suggests that cell-free hemoglobin may contribute to reperfusion injury. Faasen et al. (1988) used a simple TBARS assay and showed that the ability of hemoglobin to promote lipid peroxidation increases with storage, with incubation at 37°C, and could be minimized in the presence of the iron chelator desferrioxamine. Their experiments suggest that storage and incubation lead to the release of free iron from hemoglobin, which can then produce toxic oxygen radicals, presumably by the Haber-Weiss scheme (Halliwell and Guttridge 1989, 165).

Dawidson et al. (1988) showed that survival after reperfusion of the ischemic rat intestine with hemoglobin solutions was inferior to treatment with Ringer's lactate. These authors suggested that formation of toxic oxygen radicals could explain their rather unexpected result. The data must be regarded as inconclusive, however, because most of the in vivo studies of injury after reperfusion with hemoglobin have been done with poorly characterized solutions. We have shown recently that traces of free iron in hemoglobin preparations can promote lipid peroxidation, and other studies with well-purified solutions have shown that some of the biologic effects, such as coronary artery vasoconstriction, may be explained in part by contaminants (Macdonald et al. 1989).

Still no adequate explanation exists as to the mechanism by which iron might be liberated from heme or for the source of hydrogen peroxide in the preparations. Further studies are needed with highly purified (and characterized) hemoglobin A_0 and hemoglobin modified in various ways. The addition of cyanide ion in these experiments would also be of interest to see whether the constant interaction of oxyhemoglobin and methemoglobin could serve as a source of electrons in the Haber-Weiss reaction (Hebbel et al. 1982).

Chapter 8

The Toxicity of Hemoglobin

8.1 Early Studies on Hemoglobin Toxicity

Bayliss (1920) entitled his classic paper "Is Haemolysed Blood Toxic?" He questioned the earlier work of Paul Bert and suggested that the rabbit is an unusual animal in its sensitivity to the "fibrin-ferment" produced in clotting. He believed that the reinjection of defibrinated, lysed blood into animals was itself harmless. He went on to point out that the decreased urine output seen after hemolysis could be prevented by expansion of the plasma volume. In addition, when he injected purified stroma (red cell membranes), no toxic effects were noted. He concluded that the reduced urine output seen after hemolysis is due to osmotic effects rather than to direct toxic effects of hemoglobin or stroma. Moreover, he warned against the use of rabbits for toxicity studies because of their special sensitivity. Part of the confusion in the literature about the toxicity of hemoglobin arises from the early studies that were directed at understanding transfusion reactions.

Rabiner (Rabiner et al. 1967) showed that careful removal of red cell membranes and other impurities reduced the toxicity of hemoglobin-containing solutions. Thus, many studies carried out before 1968 may be of little more than historical value because they used relatively impure hemoglobin solutions substantially.

The central issue now, however, is whether or not hemoglobin *itself* is toxic. The question is critical because if it is, then the idea of employing it as a large-volume oxygen-carrying red cell substitute might have to be abandoned.

8.2 The Renal Toxicity of Hemoglobin Solutions

Renal toxicity is perhaps the greatest concern in the large-volume use of hemoglobin-based red cell substitutes, especially in the treatment of hemorrhagic shock. The lack of resolution of the renal toxicity problem is reflected in these statements in a 1942 textbook: "The uncertainty which apparently is the chief obstacle to utilization of hemoglobin is the question of renal damage" (Mudd 1942, 395) and "Until this question shall have been answered the use of hemoglobin as a substitute for plasma-protein must remain an academic problem" (Cannan and Redish 1942).

An important early study by Phillips et al. (1946) demonstrated that in dogs when 20–30 ml/kg blood was removed, renal blood flow ceased, whereas systolic systemic blood pressure was still 50–60 mm Hg. The flow was restored rapidly, as redistribution of blood flow favored the renal circulation. When the hemorrhage was 30–40 ml/kg, glomerular filtration also slowed, and renal circulation was not restored as the body attempted to conserve vascular volume. When hemorrhage surpassed 40–45 ml/kg or when concomitant muscle trauma occurred, maximal restriction of renal blood flow and function occurred even though the systemic systolic blood pressure did not fall below 80–100 mm Hg. Thus, in the setting of hypovolemic shock, the kidney is particularly vulnerable to toxic damage since its blood flow and function are already compromised.

In addition to the insult to the kidney from volume loss, serious renal impairment may result from hemoglobinuria associated with intravascular hemolysis or the injection of hemoglobin solutions. A voluminous literature addresses this problem, and three general theories have evolved: (1) obstruction of renal tubules by precipitation of hemoglobin or myoglobin in their lumina (Baker and Dodds 1925); (2) injury of renal tubular cells by heme pigments (Bordley 1931; DeGowin, Warner, and Randall 1938; Ayer and Gauld 1942); and (3) reduced blood flow because of vasoconstriction of renal vessels (Mason and Mann 1931; Demaria and Harris 1955). Although obstruction of tubules with precipitated hemoglobin is seen regularly in cases of massive intravascular hemolysis (Fig. 8.1), it is clear that obstruction is not needed for oliguria to occur (Oken, Arce, and Wilson 1966).

8.2.1 Contributing Factors

Dehydration and acidosis were implicated as contributing factors to the development of renal failure after hemoglobin injection in humans (Baker and Dodds 1925), but DeNavasquez (1940) could not confirm these results in rabbits. Bing (1944) felt that although acidosis did not contribute to the toxicity of oxyhemoglobin in dogs, it did potentiate the effect of methemoglobin. Hypotension (Hamilton, Hiller, and VanSlyke 1947; Rosoff and Walter 1952) and anaphylaxis (Mason and Mueller 1952) were also shown to be contributing factors.

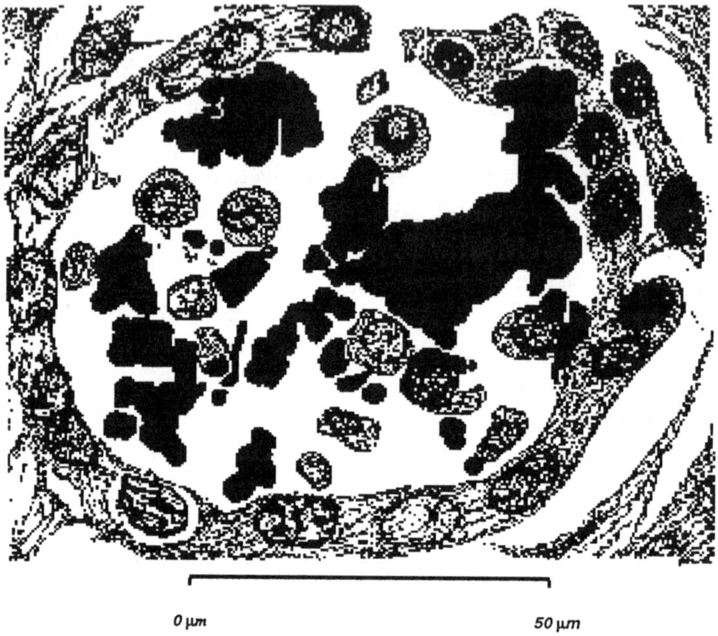

Figure 8.1. A diagram showing precipitated hemoglobin and cellular debris in a kidney tubule from an early study of blackwater fever (severe intravascular hemolysis). *Source:* Barratt and Yorke (1909), with permission.

Studies of the infusion of autologous hemoglobin in the dog have shown persistent renal failure associated with tubular obstruction (Harrison et al. 1947). Some authors reported that methemoglobin is more likely to cause renal failure than is oxyhemoglobin (Harrison et al. 1947; Bing 1944; Lalich 1952, 1955). Although dehydration and ischemia potentiate the nephrotoxic effects of hemoglobin injection (Haupt, Ochs, and Shubert 1982), they are not necessary in all cases (Goldberg 1962; Flink 1947).

The necessity of prior dehydration in the production of the hemoglobinuric renal lesion in the rat was shown by Jaenike (Jaenike 1966, 1967; Jaenike and Schneeberger 1966). Ether anesthesia, more than pentobarbital, seemed to potentiate the effect. Reduced renal blood flow occurred as soon as one hour after injection of hemoglobin but bore no particular relation to the occurrence of hematuria. At twenty-four hours inulin clearance was suppressed maximally, hemoglobin was seen in tubular lumens and vasa recta, and tubular cells appeared damaged. Recovery of function was seen at seventy-two hours, and proximal tubules were dilated, suggesting obstructive nephropathy. No compromise was observed in the normally hydrated rats.

Similarly, Maluf (1949) showed that injection of 5.8 g/kg hemolyzed red cells (equivalent to 1 liter of hemoglobin solution in a 70-kg man) into normal dogs had no effect on renal function whereas 2–3 g/kg of the hemolysate resulted in severe renal compromise with a marked drop in glomerular filtration rate, urine flow, and urine concentration. Maluf also reported that dogs in reversible histamine shock demonstrated anuria after hemoglobin solutions. Rosoff and Walter (1952) suggested further that prolonged renal anoxia is necessary to produce "hemoglobin nephrosis" in dogs.

It is clear from these considerations that demonstration of safety of new hemoglobin preparations in well-hydrated animals or human volunteers is not adequate since the large-volume use of the solutions will be primarily in shock and resuscitation, conditions in which dehydration and local tissue anoxia are likely to occur.

8.2.2 The Purity of Hemoglobin

In 1967 Rabiner and his colleagues reported a new method for the preparation of hemoglobin which made a significant impact on subsequent studies (Rabiner et al. 1967). After gentle lysis of red cells in a hypotonic phosphate buffer, the solutions were first centrifuged for ninety minutes at 16,000 x g and then for a further ninety minutes at 35,000 x g. Finally, they were passed through a 0.22-μm micropore filter. When infused into dogs, the solutions caused no adverse effects on coagulation or hemodynamics and did not form methemoglobin. No effects were seen on urea or creatinine clearance. Histologic examination of the kidneys also showed almost no adverse effects. This report has been heralded (Peskin, O'Brien, and Rabiner 1969) as a major turning point in the field, and Rabiner and his colleagues felt that they had shown that residual red cell stroma was the nephrotoxic element in previous preparations of hemoglobin solutions. Subsequent reports from Rabiner's group eliminated the centrifugation step from the preparations, without compromise of the product (Peskin, O'Brien, and Rabiner 1969; Rabiner et al. 1970).

Most workers in the field at this time were convinced that the methods of purifying hemoglobin were critical. Birndorf and Lopas, using the

Rabiner method (Birndorf, Lopas and Robboy 1971), showed that infusion of purified hemoglobin into cynomolgus monkeys was not nephrotoxic, and they then demonstrated that stroma from these solutions caused renal failure. They believed that the technique used to lyse red cells is extremely important; water lysis was discouraged because of the accumulation of membrane phospholipids which it causes (McDonald, Miller, and Roach 1951). Subsequent studies confirmed the results of Rabiner et al. (Relihan and Litwin 1972) and also showed that the renal toxicity observed after the infusion of hemoglobin into acidotic dogs was not observed when the solutions were prepared according to the "Rabiner method" (Odling-Smee and McLarnon 1984). Rabiner felt that the removal of stromal lipids was especially important in the method and stressed the use of phosphate buffer rather than water in the lysis of red cells (Rabiner 1975).

DeVenuto and co-workers (DeVenuto, Zuck, Zegna, and Moores 1977) developed a simplified method of preparing "stroma-free" hemoglobin, and they studied exchange transfusions in rats (Friedman and DeVenuto 1982). They found protein absorption droplets in proximal renal tubular cells and showed that the tubules themselves became distended with hemoglobin. The animals experienced an osmotic diuresis that resulted in dehydration and oliguria, but the authors concluded that the solutions themselves caused no permanent renal damage. Friedman and others showed subsequently that when hemoglobin was modified to increase its molecular weight and reduce its glomerular filtration, tubular obstruction did not occur (Friedman et al. 1984).

Encouraged by these results in animals, Savitsky and his co-workers infused "Rabiner" hemoglobin into human volunteers and noted a fall in urinary output and creatinine clearance, and bradycardia and hypertension (Savitsky et al. 1978). These results, along with the subsequent rumored report of adverse reactions in human recipients in an unpublished European trial, raised all of the previous fears of nephrotoxicity.

In the wake of the Savitsky clinical trials, current hemoglobin solutions were reexamined critically. The DeVenuto "crystalline" hemoglobin was found to cause decreases in platelets, rises in neutrophil counts, and a clinical picture of mild disseminated intravascular coagulation (Bolin et al. 1983).

Feola and his co-workers believed that most of the toxicity of hemoglobin solutions is due to impurities rather than to the hemoglobin molecule itself (Feola, Simoni, Canizaro, et al. 1988). They compared solutions of bovine hemoglobin prepared in various ways and studied their biologic effects in rabbits (Table 8.1). Their standard preparative procedure included filtration, chloroform treatment, removal of endotoxin with Detoxi-gel, and storage at -20°C. Table 8.1 shows that when any one of these steps was left out, significant toxicity resulted. This very interesting study points out that hemoglobin may have more than one toxic effect. Omitting the chloroform step suggests that phospholipids are toxic, lack of rigorous removal of endotoxin shows that it has a marked effect in the rabbit, and failure to store properly shows that some degradation, or polymerization in this case, might also be toxic. Note that in the table, even their best product caused drops in cell counts, a drop in fibrinogen, and complement activation.

Another attempt to prove that the toxic effects of hemoglobin can be removed by purification was carried out by Lee et al. (1989) who studied the effects of "ultrapure" polymerized bovine hemoglobin. They infused this material, with and without added bovine crude hemolysate, into rats and measured serum creatinine twenty-four hours later. They reported significant rises after the hemolysate-spiked infusions; and the rise could be controlled, to some degree, by alkalinization of the urine with bicarbonate. Unfortunately, this study does not distinguish between the effects of contaminants and unpolymerized hemoglobin, and the renal function evaluation is very limited. But similar, more extensive studies may help determine the importance of purification and chemical modification of hemoglobin.

8.2.3 The Role of Heme in Nephrotoxicity

If hemoglobin itself is toxic, it is extremely important to know what part of the molecule is responsible for toxicity. Perhaps if the molecular details of such toxicity were known, then modification could be carried out so as to prevent it. Menefee et al. (1964) found that when globin, free of heme, is administered to rats it can be identified inside renal tubular cells. They suggested that lower nephrons can become plugged after even small amounts of globin are given and that heme need not be present for hemoglobin to be toxic. Globin, however, free of heme, may be relatively insoluble and may not represent a useful model of hemoglobin toxicity.

Braun et al. (1970) studied the kinetics of the development of the renal lesion after postischemic hemoglobin infusion. They found that heme proteinuria precedes acute tubule necrosis. In kidney slices, they found that neither hemoglobin nor methemoglobin caused depressed transport in vitro, but both do when in the company of hypoxia or elevated ammonia. They also found that hematin itself depresses tubular function.

Table 8.1. Effect of Process on Hemoglobin Toxicity

Solution	I	II	III	IV	Control
<u>Process</u>					
Filtration	Yes	Yes	Yes	Yes	
Chloroform	No	Yes	Yes	Yes	
Detoxi-gel	Yes	No	Yes	Yes	
Storage	-20°C	-20°C	4°C	20°C	
<u>Clinical finding</u>					
Death	2/6	2/6	2/6	0/6	0/6
Fever	6/6	6/6	6/6	0/6	0/6
Arrhythmias	6/6	6/6	6/6	0/6	0/6
Hemoglobinuria	6/6	6/6	6/6	0/6	0/6
Hyphema	6/6	6/6	6/6	0/6	0/6
Irritability, listlessness	6/6	6/6	6/6	0/6	0/6
<u>Pathologic finding</u>					
Hemoglobin extravasation		Yes		No	No
Pulmonary edema		Yes		No	No
Hepatic congestion		Yes		Yes	No
<u>Laboratory finding</u>					
Red blood cell drop		Yes		Yes	Yes
White blood cell drop		Yes		Yes	Yes
Platelet drop		Yes		Yes	Yes
Prolonged PTT		Yes		No	No
Fibrinogen drop		Yes		Yes	Yes
Fibrin split products		Yes		No	No
C_3a rise		Yes		No	Yes
C_5a rise		Yes		No	Yes
PaO_2 drop		Yes		Yes	No
Creatinine clearance drop		Yes		Yes	No
SGPT rise		Yes		Yes	No

Source: data from Feola, Simoni, Canizaro, et al. (1988).
Note: Bovine hemoglobin was treated with glutaraldehyde and dialyzed against renal dialysis solution.

Paller and his colleagues (Paller 1988; Paller et al. 1988) showed that during reperfusion of the ischemic rat kidney reduced inulin clearance and increased urinary free iron occur. These effects could be prevented by coinfusion of desferrioxamine (an iron chelator) during the first sixty minutes of reperfusion. Notably, inulin-conjugated desferrioxamine was much more effective than dextran-conjugated desferrioxamine, suggesting that tubular cells are the site of damage of free iron since dextran-conjugated desferrioxamine is not filtered by the glomerulus.

8.2.4 Colloid Osmotic Pressure

It is possible that the colloid osmotic pressure (COP) of hemoglobin could play a role in nephrotoxicity. This colloid osmotic pressure opposes hydrostatic pressure, the driving force for glomerular filtration within the glomerular capillaries. Thus, if the colloid osmotic pressure of the plasma is increased, the glomerular filtration rate would be expected to decrease on this basis alone. This probably explains why patients who receive massive infusions of albumin may become oliguric or even anuric (Rozich and Paul 1989). Acute renal failure may occur in sepsis, hypotension, or exposure to nephrotoxic substances and may lead to diminished renal blood flow, further reducing the hydrostatic pressure. Cell-free hemoglobin could be used in any of these clinical settings.

The expected colloid osmotic pressure can be calculated on the basis of the plasma protein concentration (Nitta et al. 1981), but the relationships will be different for hemoglobin modified in different ways. A controversy exists as to what the optimal molecular size of cell-free hemoglobin should be, and its oncotic effect will be a strong determinant in the eventual formulations.

8.3 Liver Toxicity

Friedman and others found that when rats were exchange transfused with unmodified hemoglobin solutions to 75 percent of their initial blood volume they survived but exhibited a centrilobular hepatic necrosis (Friedman et al. 1978). They found that they could prevent the necrosis by additional administration of hemoglobin solution (DeVenuto, Friedman, and Mellick 1980) and concluded that the liver insult was caused by hypovolemia and liver hypoxia consequent to anemia as hemoglobin was cleared from the circulation. These workers showed subsequently that pyridoxylated, polymerized hemoglobin could be used for exchange transfusions in rats, and they could find no evidence of hepatic necrosis

(Friedman, et al. 1984). These studies are reassuring but were carried out in only one species. Concerns about hepatic toxicity in other animals, especially rabbits, were raised by Feola (Feola, Simoni, Canizaro, et al. 1988) and White (White, Murray, Greene, Smith, et al. 1986).

A different modified hemoglobin, cross-linked between α chains with the reagent bis(3,5-dibromosalicyl)fumarate (DBBF) (see Chapter 5), was studied in rats and pigs at the Letterman Army Institute of Research. The rats were given bolus injections of hyperoncotic solutions containing 14 g/dl hemoglobin at 40, 50, and 60 percent of initial blood volume, and liver histology was studied after forty-eight hours. Hepatic lesions were found only where the dose was high enough to cause pulmonary edema and were also seen in animals given equivalent doses of albumin (Clifford, Wessels, and Smith 1989). Four pigs received 72 ml/kg modified hemoglobin, and the histology was examined at 1, 4, 7, and 15 days after transfusion (Fig. 8.2). A fifth pig received 100 ml/kg and was killed 7.5 hours after the procedure. At 7.5 hours, hepatocytes were vacuolated, and by day 1, mild centrolobular necrosis was seen. By day 4 modest numbers of inflammatory cells were seen in the centrolobular zone, but these were fewer by day 7, and by day 15 the liver lobules were normal (Smith, Schuschereba, et al. 1990).

Although examination of liver histology should be a part of the evaluation of any proposed red cell substitute solution, care must be exercised not to confuse species differences and the effects of contaminants with the effects of hemoglobin. In addition, it is clear from these studies that hemoglobin solutions can produce histologic abnormalities as a result of their oncotic, oxygen-carrying, and possibly direct toxic effects.

8.4 Neurotoxicity

Although renal and other toxicity of hemoglobin solutions has been well studied (if not well understood), the effects of such solutions on the brain and nervous system may be of paramount concern. Fears of neurotoxicity arise from the knowledge that nervous tissue is rich in lipid and may be subject to peroxidation with resultant formation of oxygen radicals. Although the blood-brain barrier is a potent mechanism that protects from such effects, if the barrier breaks down for any reason nervous tissue could be at risk.

Studies done at the Letterman Army Institute of Research by Schuschereba and his co-workers (1983) showed that 75 percent exchange transfusions in rats using unmodified hemoglobin led to retinal axonal damages. Subsequent studies by O'Mara et al. (1978) were designed to show whether infusion of hemoglobin solutions affected the ability of rats to perform a prelearned task. The results showed that such animals could not perform a bar-pressing task after 65–75 percent exchange transfusion with unmodified hemoglobin.

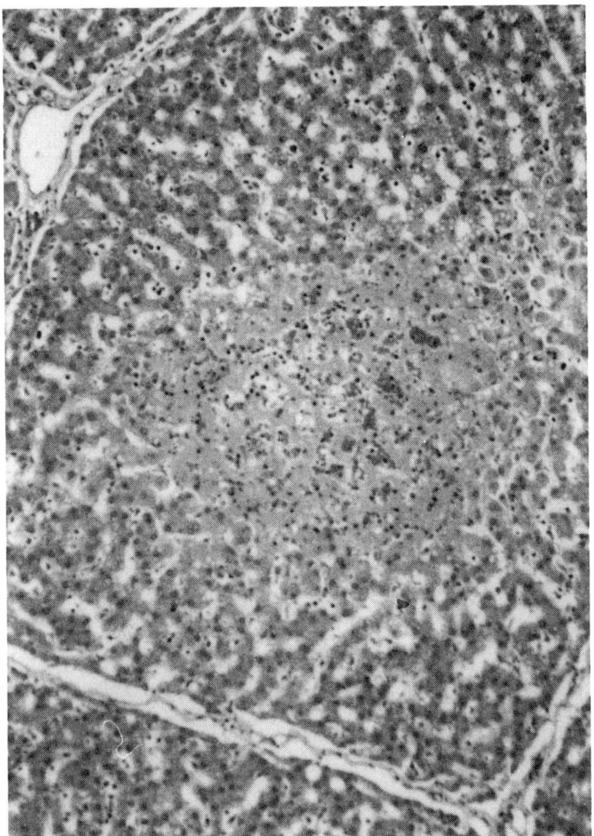

Figure 8.2. Centrolobular necrosis in the pig after a total red cell exchange transfusion with hemoglobin cross-linked between the α chains with bis(3,5-dibromosalicyl)fumarate ($\alpha\alpha$-Hb). The extent of the lesion varies among animals but is always self-limited.

We felt the studies by Schuschereba, O'Mara and their co-workers were extremely important and, if verified, could limit further development of hemoglobin-based red cell substitutes. Thus, new studies were designed using αα-cross-linked hemoglobin prepared by the best methods available. The solutions were prepared free of endotoxin, and the rats were trained to negotiate a rather complicated water maze. Two studies were undertaken. In the first, 20 ml/kg of a 14 g/dl solution of cross-linked hemoglobin solution was infused into rats, and their ability to negotiate the maze was evaluated (Przybelski et al. 1989). No degradation of performance whatever was noted. The second study (Przybelski et al. 1990) was similar except the rats were subjected to a 50 percent hemorrhage prior to resuscitation with the cross-linked hemoglobin. Again, no degradation in performance was noted. In addition, some of the animals resuscitated with Ringer's lactate died. No brain pathology was noted in the αα-hemoglobin animals either after treatment or 10 days later, but lesions were present in 25 percent of the animals resuscitated with Ringer's lactate.

These results were extremely important to us because they indicated that if hemoglobin is purified and cross-linked it need not be toxic to the nervous system. Much more work in this area needs to be done, however, because we still lack an explanation for the toxicity in the original studies. For example, the Schuschereba and O'Mara experiments were done with unmodified hemoglobin, which might have crossed the blood-brain barrier. Some injuries, such as shock, infection, or trauma, could result in a breakdown of the blood-brain barrier, and toxicity could result.

8.5 Incompatible Transfusion Reactions

Transfusion of incompatible blood has been used as a model for the study of hemoglobin toxicity since it often results in massive hemolysis. Typically, patients develop a subjective sense of restlessness and anxiety followed by flushing, tachycardia, fever, chills, and sometimes dull, aching pain in the back and thighs. Precordial pain, nausea, and vomiting may also occur. The temperature may reach 105° F, and delirium may ensue.

A hemorrhagic tendency may develop, and blood may ooze from the transfusion site and the mucous membranes. Fibrinogen and other clotting factors may be depleted, probably as a result of fibrin formation after liberation of thromboplastic substances. Thrombocytopenia and leukopenia may also be found.

The blood plasma turns red immediately after the transfusion begins, and the urine turns dark as hemoglobin is cleared. In severe reactions, renal failure occurs. Anuria can develop rapidly and subside after twenty-four hours, only to be followed by progressive uremia. If the reaction is not too severe, diuresis and recovery occur after several days; however, death can occur as late as the seventh to nineteenth day, and diuresis and recovery can occur as late as the sixteenth day. Severe cases of renal failure must be treated with potent diuretics, or even hemodialysis.

8.5.1 Stroma versus Hemoglobin

Reid (1929) showed that after intravascular hemolysis in dogs, the volume of the kidney, measured plethysmographically, decreased, indicating a drop in blood flow to the organ. Later, Mason and Mann (1931) attempted to determine whether this effect was caused by the stroma of hemolyzed red cells or hemoglobin. They found a more pronounced effect with hemoglobin than with stroma and concluded that stroma had no effect on renal blood flow and function.

Schmidt and Holland (1967) used incompatible stroma injections in two antibody-forming patients to absorb antibody in preparation for life-saving surgery for which transfusion of incompatible units was highly likely. They prepared stroma from the blood of multiple incompatible donors and administered the suspensions intravenously. The resulting reaction was characterized by a drop in urine output, systemic *hypotension*, and marked granulocytopenia with rebound. Their previous experience (Shulman et al. 1965) had shown that *compatible* stroma injection is innocuous, and they concluded that incompatible transfusion reactions were due to the involvement of antibody-antigen complexes, not simply stromal components.

These observations contrast with the clinical effects of hemoglobin injections: although decreased urine output also occurs, *hypertension* is the rule (Savitsky et al. 1978). Thus, both hemoglobin and stroma seem to cause oliguria or even anuria, but other systemic effects are perhaps different. This may explain some of the confusion in the literature.

8.5.2 Distilled Water Injections

Useful information about the toxic effects of hemoglobin comes from the study of distilled water injections. Such experiments were carried out to understand the effects of acute, massive hemolysis as occurs, for example, in blackwater fever, and to illustrate the effects of *compatible* stroma.

Blackburn et al. (1954) infused distilled water into ten volunteers. Five experienced fever and mild backache about twenty minutes after the infusion. Oliguria occurred in seven of the ten, and in four of these urine flow ceased for a short time. Renal plasma flow dropped severely, and renal vascular resistance rose in six of the seven patients who had oliguria, suggesting renal arterial vasoconstriction. The authors noted the similarity of these findings to those seen after infusion of stroma-free hemoglobin. However, some of the subjects who had hemoglobinuria had no renal effects. Moreover, there were no significant changes in systemic blood pressure or pulse rate. These studies seem to indicate that hemolysis of compatible blood may cause renal vasoconstriction due to hemoglobin, not stroma.

Blackburn et al. (1954) concluded that water infusions cause oliguria in some patients without systemic cardiovascular effects and that oliguria is probably caused by renal vasoconstriction. The renal damage in their patients was reversible, responding to a volume load (mannitol) and renal vasodilator (parathyroid hormone). They believed that renal vasoconstriction could lead to severe renal ischemia in the presence of mild to moderate shock, and this could explain their variable results.

A curious feature of these data on water infusions is that not all subjects react to the same extent. This is illustrated by the experience with transurethral resection of the prostate, in which distilled water is used to irrigate the bladder. Landsteiner and Finch (1947), after observing a fatality, found that ten of fifteen patients undergoing routine procedures had evidence of hemolysis, three with very high levels of plasma hemoglobin, but only one had temporary oliguria.

8.6 "Crush" Syndrome

The association of myoglobinuria and renal injury was established in 1940 with the recognition that patients whose limbs had been crushed by debris in the London Blitz and who recovered from the initial shock often develped renal failure (Bywaters and Beall 1940). This was called the *crush syndrome*, and was studied subsequently in detail by Corcoran and Page (1945). These authors injected hemoglobin, myoglobin, and hematin (sodium ferrihemate) into acidotic dogs and observed an analog to the crush syndrome. Of particular interest, they found that hematin was particularly toxic, causing renal vasoconstriction and cellular toxicity.

A model of the crush syndrome is the intramuscular injection of glycerol, which causes myoglobinemia and myoglobinuria. Paller used this model to show that when iron chelators are present the renal damage from glycerol injection is minimized (Paller 1988). However, Grisham (1985) has shown that oxymyoglobin is more effective as a catalyst for the peroxidation of arachidonic acid than is metmyoglobin or hemoglobin. It would be interesting to correlate the propensity of different hemoglobin solutions to cause renal damage with their propensity for hemeglobin dissociation.

8.7 Macrophage and Neutrophil Stimulation

An intriguing possible explanation for some of the diverse consequences of hemoglobin infusions is the elaboration of the arachidonic acid metabolites, the thromboxanes, known to be produced by platelets and macrophages as well as in the kidney (Miyamoto et al. 1988; Morrison 1986). Thromboxane A_2 is a potent vasoconstrictor and has been shown to be produced in the kidney after glycerol injection to induce renal failure (Benabe et al. 1980; Morrison, Benabe, and Hoffman 1980).

As mentioned above, subcutaneous glycerol may induce renal failure by a mechanism thought to involve liberation of heme pigments from muscle. In the rat, direct infusion of the stable derivative of thromboxane A_2 (thromboxane B_2) reduces the glomerular filtration rate by increasing renal vascular resistance (Baylis 1987). Although thromboxane may play no role in regulating the glomerular filtration rate in normal humans (Zipser 1985) thromboxane A_2 synthesis in the nephrotic syndrome is increased and may be responsible for increasing the basement membrane permeability to protein (Remuzzi et al. 1985).

In conscious rats (Rabinovici, Rudolph, and Feuerstein 1989) and sheep (Miyamoto et al. 1988), infusion of liposomes leads almost immediately to increased mean arterial pressure and heart rate, decreased platelet counts, and increased thromboxanes. These effects were short-lived, and all measured values returned to baseline by about 120 minutes. The authors of these studies speculated that the liposome particles interacted with platelets and leukocytes to generate the humoral vasoconstrictors.

Thromboxane A_2 may play an important role in the development of endotoxin shock, a situation in which hemoglobin could be used in large quantities. Improved survival of rats (Fukumoto and Tanaka 1983) and sheep (Cumming et al. 1989) has been demonstrated after administering thromboxane A_2 inhibitors prior to endotoxin.

Of further interest, some preparations of perfluorocarbons have similar effects. FC-43 (perfluorotributylamine, 25 percent, weight/volume) emulsified with Pluronic F-68 (polyoxypropylene-polyoxyethylene copolymer, 3.2 percent, weight/volume) was shown by Bucala, Kowakami, and Cerami (1983) to be cytotoxic to macrophages in vitro. The authors speculated that the mechanism of this toxicity could be that the emulsion particles (0.1 μm diameter) may be taken up by phagocytic cells. Inside the cell, the high oxygen delivered could be toxic if the normal celluar mechanisms of detoxifying oxygen free radicals were overwhelmed. To support this concept, the same authors also reported that when incubations of FC-43 and macrophages were carried out in the presence of low oxygen pressure, toxicity appeared to be less.

It is possible that some of the reported toxic effects of hemoglobin solutions could be explained by similar mechanisms, particularly if they are contaminated with phospholipid or if the hemoglobin molecules are polymerized to a degree that they may stimulate phagocytic cells (Pristoupil, Kramlova, and Marik 1989).

Perhaps many of these observations can be drawn together with the unifying hypothesis that they all involve stimulation of macrophages such as those found in the pulmonary vascular tree (pulmonary interstitial macrophages). These cells are present in the pulmonary vascular trees of many animals but to varying extents. Norman Staub, in whose laboratory much of the recent important work in this area has been done, found that all species of the mammalian order Artiodactyla (even-toed, cloven-hooved) contain such cells (Staub 1988). These animals show marked but transient pulmonary hypertension after even very small injections of particulate dyes, liposomes, foreign blood cells, endotoxin, and bacteria. In contrast, members of three other mammalian orders (Rodentia, Lagomorpha, and Carnivora) are unresponsive (Miyamoto, Schultz, and Staub 1977; Miyamoto et al. 1987). These results also underscore the importance of animal model selection in carrying out studies of toxic effects of red cell substitutes.

Recent work has suggested that neutrophil stimulation is important in organ injury associated with ischemia and shock. These cells can be stimulated to produce a glycoprotein that mediates adherence to endothelial cell surfaces (Vedder et al. 1989). If hemoglobin or a contaminant in hemoglobin solutions also stimulates these cells, toxicity of some of the preparations may be explained.

8.8 Complement Activation

The activation of complement and the stimulation of procoagulant activity have been reported with native unmodified, cross-linked, and pyridoxylated-polymerized hemoglobin. A study by Wilson and Thomas (1979) showed that unmodified hemoglobin prepared from either normal or sickle-cell red cells activated C_3 conversion when the hemoglobin concentration was greater than 1.5 g/dl. However, preparations of stroma from the same blood samples or from buffy coats did not. These authors were concerned primarily with patients with chronic hemolytic anemia, such as sickle-cell disease, and speculated that if the complement system is overwhelmed by massive hemolysis, defective opsonization of bacteria, especially *Pneumococcus* and *Salmonella*, could result. The clinical significance of these properties is not yet clear, nor are their mechanisms. In addition, preliminary experiments from our laboratory have indicated that perhaps modified hemoglobin solutions can bind to endotoxin in some specific manner (White, Murray, Smith, et al. 1986). If this proves to be true, infusion of the materials could aggravate sepsis and the effects of endotoxin.

8.9 Vasoconstriction

8.9.1 Coronary Vasoconstriction

Hemoglobin solutions are known to be vasoactive. As early as 1900, Brodie showed that a crude hemolysate, infused into cats, caused a fall in blood pressure and heart rate (Brodie 1900). However, Amberson later showed that this immediate fall in blood pressure is followed by a rise (Amberson et al. 1934–35). More recently, Moss and co-workers found that stroma-free hemoglobin raises blood pressure but reduces heart rate in primates (Moss et al. 1976), effects noted earlier by Savitsky in humans (Savitsky et al. 1978). Gould and co-workers also found a rise in pulmonary artery pressure and resistance during exchange transfusions (Gould et al. 1986).

These effects have not found in vitro models that shed light on the basic mechanisms. Thus, Vogel and co-workers (Vogel et al. 1988) reported that both stroma-free and pyridoxylated hemoglobins cause coronary vasoconstriction in the isolated, perfused rabbit heart. Glutaraldehyde cross-linked hemoglobin, bovine hemoglobin purified by high pressure liquid chromatography (HPLC) (Vogel et al. 1988), or human hemoglobin purified using either ATP-affinity chromatography (Hsia and Song S 1988) or HPLC (Macdonald et al. 1989) also seem to be free of the vasoconstrictor activity in the isolated, perfused heart.

Macdonald and co-workers showed that hemoglobin A_0, produced in our laboratory, did not cause coronary vasoconstriction in a similar model, nor did αα-cross-linked hemoglobin; but stroma-free hemoglobin did (Macdonald et al. 1989). These findings agree with those of Lieberthal et al. (1989). Moreover, Macdonald has also observed that prior perfusion of a coronary bed with methemoglobin seems to abolish the subsequent vasoconstrictor activity of a solution of stroma-free hemoglobin, known to be vasoconstrictive in a nonpreconditioned heart (Macdonald 1989). This puzzling observation remains to be explained.

Gilroy et al. (1989) attempted to elucidate the vasoconstrictor effect by studying different preparations of hemoglobin (Table 8.2). The materials studied included pyridoxylated, polymerized hemoglobin prepared by

Table 8.2. Effect of Purification Method on Vasoconstrictor Activity

	DV	G	C	PR	PR
	Glut Dial	Glut Dial	Glut Dial		Dial
Hemoglobin (g/dl)	10 –13	10–13	10–13		
Methemoglobin (%)	15–27	8–18	5–13		
Phospholipid (mg/dl)	6–15	3–5	1–2		
dP (mm Hg)20.6	2.0 ±2.2	33.5	23.6 ±18.7	20.6	7.6

Source: data from Gilroy et al. (1989). Note: The abbreviations used are: DV: DeVenuto (crystallization); G: Greenburg (ultracentrifugation); C: Chloroform extraction; PR: pure red cells (filtered to remove white blood cells and platelets); dP: pressure rise (vasoconstriction); Glut: glutaraldehyde; Dial: dialysis. Standard deviations are shown if available.

chloroform extraction, ultracentrifugation, or crystallization, along with hemoglobin prepared from purified (platelet and white-cell poor) red cells. They concluded from their studies that dialysis is important in reducing vasoconstriction in glutaraldehyde-treated hemoglobin. However, as Table 8.2 shows, the vasoconstrictor effect is consistent with Macdonald's results in which methemoglobin seems to prevent vasoconstriction.

In the in situ perfused dog heart, Biro found that unmodified hemolysate caused coronary vasoconstriction whereas partially purified hemolysate and pyridoxylated, polymerized hemoglobin had much less activity (Biro et al. 1988). However, in these preparations, infusion of adenosine, which normally increases flow by vasodilatation, had no effect; that is, they were maximally vasoconstricted (and probably hypoxic) to start. Purified, pyridoxylated hemoglobin polyethylene conjugate (PHP) also has less vasoconstrictor activity than unmodified hemoglobin in the isolated rat heart (Yamakawa et al. 1990).

Definitive identification of the vasoactive component(s) has not yet been made, but it is likely that this model system may yield important information about the mechanism of vasoconstriction observed with hemoglobin solutions. However, if the mechanism is mediated by products of other cells, such as macrophages, then this model may not provide the needed answers. For example, Salari and Walker (1989) stimulated rat peritoneal macrophages with endotoxin and perfused rat hearts with Krebs medium that had been exposed to the macrophages. These cells released substances that were vasoactive in the coronary circulation. Thus, perfusion of a heart with a completely cell-free solution may not be as useful a model as perfusion with a blood/hemoglobin mixture.

How endothelial cells transmit signals to adjacent smooth muscle cells is under intense study in a variety of disease states. In addition to chemical stimuli, hyperosmotic solutions as well as certain mechanical stimuli can cause relaxation of smooth muscle (Munakata, Mitzner, and Menkes 1988). In addition, all or a part of the vasoconstrictor effect of hemoglobin might be explained by its known ability to bind nitric oxide (NO), the putative endothelial-derived relaxing factor (EDRF). It is quite possible that solution of the vasoconstrictor problem might also provide new basic information about the regulation of vascular tone.

8.9.2 Pulmonary Vasoconstriction

Hemoglobin solutions have also been reported to cause vasoconstriction in the pulmonary circulation. White, Murray, Greene, et al. (1986) infused unmodified hemoglobin solutions into rabbits and found, on microscopic examination of the lungs, evidence of microthrombi formation, suggesting antemortem pulmonary hypertension. Mohanty et al. (1989) also discovered microscopic evidence for pulmonary hypertension in rabbits but found a relationship between the extent of toxicity and the rate of infusion. Although not conclusive, these observations are consistent with the above suggestion that these hemoglobin solutions could have stimulated cytokine release from macrophages. Further studies are needed to understand the unusual sensitivity of rabbits in these experiments.

8.10 Activated Oxygen

The term *activated oxygen* refers to powerful oxidizing agents such as superoxide ($O_2^{\cdot}$), peroxide H_2O_2, hydroxyl free radical ($HO^{\cdot}$), and singlet oxygen ($O_2^{=}$). Some of these, such as superoxide, are dismuted very effectively by superoxide dismutase, which is present in high concentration in many tissues. Others, such as hydroxyl free radical, are extremely difficult to measure and quantitate because they are powerful oxidizing agents and react quickly. Formation of these reactive oxygen molecules is essential for many cellular functions such as bacteria killing by phagocytes and the selective killing of many tumor cells. However, in certain settings, they can cause destruction of normal tissue.

In humans, red cell membranes are freely permeable to oxygen and hydrogen peroxide, and the redox system GSSG/GSH reduces these toxic molecules in hemorrhagic or endotoxin shock or in other types of oxidative stress (Nemeth and Boda 1989). Thus, human red cells may have an important role as scavengers of extracellular hydrogen peroxide and may play a role in protection from oxidative damage.

For oxygen free radicals to cause tissue damage, three biochemical conditions must be involved (Saltman 1989): (1) oxygen must be present under conditions in which it can accept reducing equivalents and protons to form hydrogen peroxide with or without superoxide; (2) a target molecule must be present which binds a redox active molecule, most often iron or copper; and (3) hydrogen peroxide must interact with the reduced metal to generate hydroxyl free radicals that carry out the actual oxidation or tissue damage.

Faasen et al. (1988) suggested that hemoglobin itself could promote the production of activated oxygen and hydroxyl radicals, and the infusion of hemoglobin into the intact animal may present a serious oxidative stress that could overwhelm natural defenses. There are several mechanisms whereby this could occur, but none of them has been proven. First, the solution itself could contain free iron that could react with hydrogen peroxide to produce hydroxyl radicals. Whether or not iron leaves the heme group is controversial: in vivo the affinity of transferrin for free iron is so high that it is unlikely that free iron would be detected. Second, free iron from other sources could accumulate in the animal in hemorrhagic shock, making this the most potentially dangerous clinical application (Mazur, Baez, and Shorr 1955). Third, the preparations could contain activated lipid peroxides, which themselves could peroxidate host lipids in a chain reaction that could lead to serious tissue damage. Unfortunately, too few data are available to address the degree of this problem.

If activated radicals do cause tissue toxicity, however, there is hope that remedies can be devised since chelators, reducing enzymes, and free radical scavengers could be protective in certain instances (Hedlund 1988). This consideration is particularly important in the resuscitation setting since the reperfusion of ischemic tissue is exactly where a resupply of oxygen could lead to significant generation of radicals.

8.11 Reperfusion Injury

Patients who undergo even transient ischemia, either local or global, are prone to consequent organ damage. Perhaps the most devastating and least reversible of these is cerebral hypoxia and resultant brain damage. Postischemic renal failure is also common and is easier to quantitate and study. For many years the etiology of this lesion was thought to be hypoxia.

More recently it has been appreciated that the insult occurs when oxygen is resupplied and toxic oxygen radicals are generated. Oxygen radicals have been implicated in renal reperfusion injury (McCord 1985) and a number of other disease states as well (Halliwell and Gutteridge 1984). This general area has come to be known as *reperfusion injury,* and new insights have been gained from the realization that toxic radicals form when oxygen is resupplied to ischemic tissue. Reperfusion injury is an extremely important consideration in the design of resuscitation fluids because the proposal has been made that hemoglobin poses an additional oxidant stress (Faasen et al. 1988).

Another source of oxygen radicals is the degradation of hypoxanthine to uric acid by the enzyme xanthine oxidase. This enzyme is normally a dehydrogenase, but in response to global ischemia it is converted to an oxygenase. In the rat, this conversion is presumed to proceed by proteolytic alteration of the dehydrogenase with half-times of 3.6, 6, 7, and 14 hours (at 37^oC) for liver, kidney, heart, and lung, respectively (Engerson et al. 1984).

During ischemia, hypoxanthine, a substrate for hypoxanthine oxygenase, accumulates in certain tissues as a result of breakdown of ATP (Fig. 8.3). When hydrogen peroxide is produced according to the Haber-

Weiss reaction, hydroxyl radicals may be formed:

$$H_2O_2 + O_2^- \longrightarrow O_2 + HO^- + HO^{\cdot} \qquad (1)$$

In aqueous solution, this reaction has a rate constant approaching zero, but it is catalyzed by transition metal ions including iron and copper. Thus, the full scheme becomes

$$Fe^{3+} + O_2^- \longrightarrow Fe^{2+} + O_2 \qquad (2)$$

$$Fe^{2+} + H_2O_2 \longrightarrow Fe^{3+} + HO^{\cdot} + HO^- \qquad (3)$$

(Fenton reaction)

$$O_2^- + H_2O_2 \longrightarrow O_2 + HO^{\cdot} + HO^- \qquad (4)$$

(net reaction)

This role for free iron to catalyze the Haber-Weiss scheme by acting as a Fenton reagent is difficult to demonstrate because only trace amounts of reactants are required. Much of the evidence for its participation is indirect such as the inhibition of hydroxyl radical formation in the presence of the iron chelator desferrioxamine as shown by Gutteridge, Richmond, and Halliwell (1979).

8.11.1 Lipid Peroxidation

Lipid peroxidation is a chain reaction leading to a broad spectrum of tissue damage. Reduced iron compounds react with lipid hydroperoxides to give alkoxy radicals:

$$\begin{aligned} &Lipid-O_2H + Fe^{2+}-complex \longrightarrow \\ &\quad Fe^{3+}-complex + HO^{\cdot} + Lipid-O^{\cdot} \end{aligned} \qquad (5)$$

Peroxy radicals are formed in the presence of Fe^{3+}:

$$Lipid-O_2 + Fe^{3+}-complex \longrightarrow Lipid-O^{\cdot} + H^{+} + Fe^{2+}-complex \quad (6)$$

Both peroxy and alkoxy radicals can stimulate the lipid peroxidation chain reaction. All unsaturated fatty acids contain lipid hydroperoxides.

Although it is clear that iron participates in this reaction, the initiation of lipid peroxidation by iron probably requires some product of ferrous autooxidation; that is, Fe^{2+} or Fe^{3+} alone or the mere presence of activated oxygen radicals is not sufficient to initiate the reaction. It is likely that a ferrous-dioxygen-ferric chelate complex is the species that initiates the reaction (Bucher, Ming, and Aust 1983).

8.11.2 The Source of H_2O_2 and O_2^-

Any biologic system that produces O_2^- will produce hydrogen peroxide by the dismutase reaction:

$$2O_2^- + 2H^+ \longrightarrow H_2O_2 + O_2 \quad (7)$$

The rate of formation of hydrogen peroxide by this mechanism is dependent on oxygen concentration (hence oxygen toxicity at very high oxygen tensions) and is faster at lower pH. Hydrogen peroxide production by this mechanism has been found in bacteria, spermatozoa, and other organisms. Many enzymes, including glycolate and urate oxidases (xanthine oxidase), produce hydrogen peroxide without intermediate O_2^- (Halliwell and Gutteridge 1984).

8.11.3 The Occurrence of Xanthine Oxidase

A test of the hypothetical importance of xanthine oxidase in the pathogenesis of reperfusion injury is the use of the drug allopurinol, a competitive inhibitor of xanthine oxidase. As reviewed by Cohen (1989), trials of this drug were surprisingly ineffective in controlling infarct size after coronary occlusion in the dog. Recently, it has been shown that the conversion of xanthine dehydrogenase to oxidase is barely detectable after one hour of ischemia and is only 50 percent complete after seven hours in the rat heart (Engerson et al. 1987). Since this is an extremely active area of current research, the importance of xanthine oxidase in reperfusion injury will undoubtedly become clear in the near future.

8.11.4 Source of Iron

Approximately 4 g of iron is present in the normal human body. However, there is virtually no free iron in human serum because Fe^{3+} is transported bound to transferrin, available for synthesis of hemoglobin and other enzymes. The affinity constant for iron by this protein is approximately 10^{23}. Ferritin iron is a second storage form, not normally available for biologic reactions. Apoferritin binds Fe^{2+} but oxidizes it to Fe^{3+}. Free iron has been detected in synovial and cerebrospinal fluids (Halliwell and Gutteridge 1984). Although copper can also act as a Fenton reagent, typically only 80 mg is present in the human body.

Whether the scheme shown in Figure 8.3 occurs in reperfusion injury depends on the presence of free iron for the formation of $HO^{\cdot}$ radicals. Mazur noted that free iron increases and transferrin saturation decreases during hemorrhagic shock in the dog (Fig. 8.4) (Mazur, Baez, and Shorr 1955). Later this group went on to show, by giving purine substrates, that hepatic ferritin iron can be released into plasma after reduction by xanthine oxidase (Mazur et al. 1958). Thus, a modern version of their proposed mechanism includes the conversion of xanthine dehydrogenase to xanthine oxidase, accumulation of purine substrates during hypoxia, resupply of oxygen, and then the release of Fe^{3+} from ferritin stores. This iron would then be available to act as a Fenton reagent.

Paller and co-workers showed that urinary iron increases in the reperfusion period (Paller 1988; Paller et al. 1988). They also showed that the decrease in inulin clearance and the increase in lipid peroxidation normally seen after ischemia of the kidney could be prevented when the reperfusate contained the iron chelator desferrioxamine. They also showed that the prevention of injury was more effective if desferrioxamine is conjugated to inulin, which is cleared by the kidney, than to dextran, which is not.

8.11.5 Protective Mechanisms

Superoxide dismutase is a copper-containing enzyme (formerly known as erythrocuperin) in the red cell. It is ubiquitous in aerobic organisms and is known to convert two molecules of $O_2^{\cdot -}$ to oxygen and hydrogen peroxide (Misra and Fridovich 1972). Hydrogen peroxide is broken down to oxygen and water by catalase and, within the red cell, is reduced by reduced glutathione, catalyzed by glutathione peroxidase. The resultant oxidized glutathione is reduced by NADPH from the pentose pathway. Finally, additional defense against oxidation is provided by vitamin E, which protects against $O_2^{\cdot -}$ and hydrogen peroxide. These mechanisms are not available to cell-free hemoglobin. The enzymes could be packaged in liposomes with hemoglobin, an approach that has interested some workers in the field of red cell substitutes.

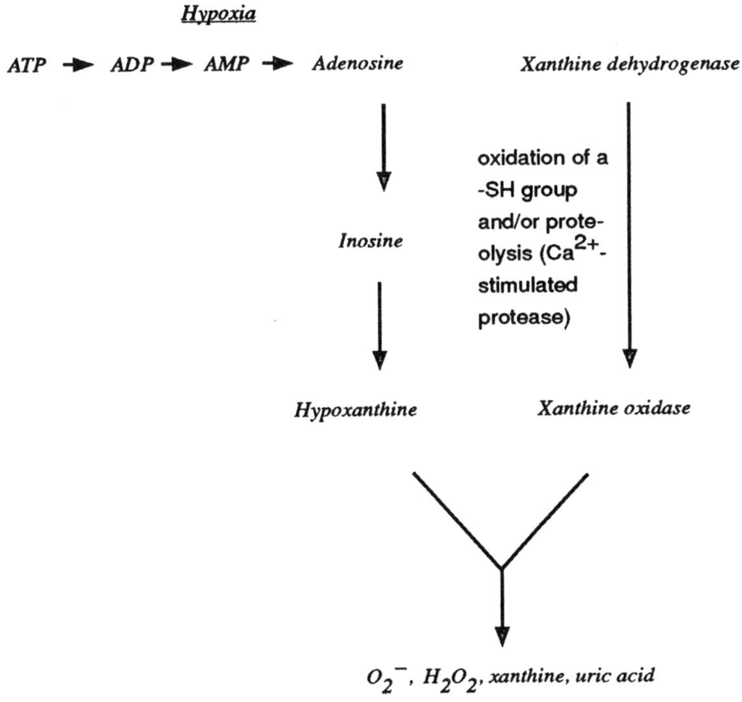

Figure 8.3. Xanthine-xanthine oxidase reactions. Under conditions of hypoxia and ischemia, hypoxanthine accumulates and xanthine dehydrogenase becomes an oxidase. When O_2 is resupplied, oxygen radicals may be formed. *Source:* adapted from McCord (1967).

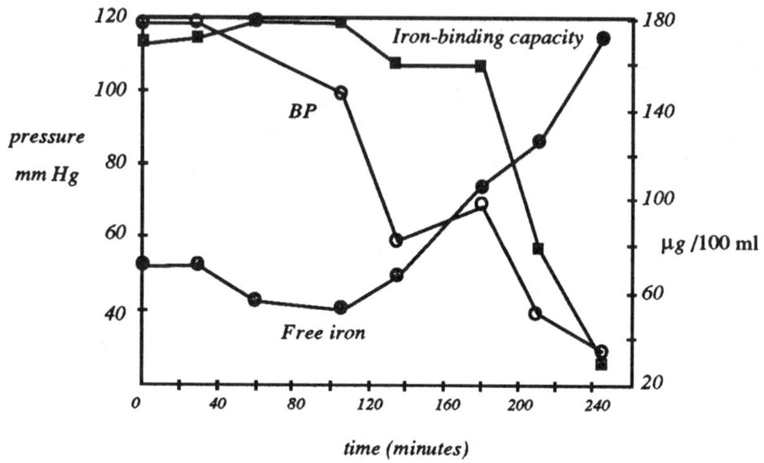

Figure 8.4. Plasma iron during hemorrhage in the dog. *BP*, blood pressure. *Source:* adapted from Mazur, Baez, and Shorr (1955).

8.12 Immunogenicity

The infusion of large quantities of protein solution into a recipient raises the fear that antibodies may be formed which might lead to immune reactions. Although hemoglobin is weakly immunogenic, very specific antibodies have been prepared for the detection of hemoglobin mutants. Chang and Varma (1988) showed that heterologous infusions of hemoglobin lead to higher antibody titers than do homologous infusions, and the more highly derivatized preparations are more likely to be immunogenic. Still, to obtain any immune response at all, their experiments required the use of adjuvants. The clinical consequences of these observations remain to be understood, but the issue is extremely important if animal hemoglobin is to be used. It will be critical to know whether repeated administration of hemoglobin to human subjects will result in immunization.

8.13 Coagulation Defects

Some natural and synthetic plasma expanders cause hemostatic problems. Coagulation defects have been demonstrated either in vivo or in vitro with dextran, hydroxyethyl starch, polyvinylpyrrolidone, gelatin, and some polyamino acids. Alexander et al. (1975) suggested that these problems are caused by the complexing of certain coagulation factors and diminished platelet function. Thus, suspicion is justifiably raised concerning the effect of modified hemoglobin solutions and particularly those that involve conjugation of hemoglobin to one of the other plasma expanders mentioned above.

Birndorff, Lopas, and Robboy (1971), after showing that infusion of highly purified hemoglobin was safe in a series of cynomolgus monkeys, injected purified stroma into a separate series of monkeys. They observed disseminated intravascular coagulation, as demonstrated by depressed platelet counts, fibrinogen and factors II, VIII, and V concentrations, activation of fibrinolysis, and lengthening of the prothrombin and partial thromboplastin times. Autopsies of these animals revealed hemorrhagic pulmonary and renal infarctions. Cochin et al. (1972) reported that red cell stroma, but not hemoglobin itself, caused drops in platelet counts, elevated phospholipid concentration, and prolonged coagulation times in rabbits. Coagulation defects have not been demonstrated in rats infused with 10 percent blood volume of either unmodified or polymerized human or rat hemoglobin (Ning and Chang 1990).

Few data on stimulation of platelet function are available. Lalla, Ning, and Chang (1989) reported that neither purified human hemoglobin nor pyridoxylated, polymerized hemoglobin had a significant effect on ADP-induced platelet aggregation. This would seem to be a necessary requirement for any prospective red cell substitute preparation.

Smith and Winslow (1991) studied the effects of hemoglobin, modified and unmodified, on the procoagulant activity of mononuclear cells. They found that hematin, methemoglobin, and hemoglobin all elicited a procoagulant response in peripheral blood mononuclear cells and activated complement; isolated globin had none of these effects. Whether or not the procoagulant material is the same as tissue thromboplastin was not established, but this could be an important point since the latter has been found to be elevated for many days in postsurgical patients (Blakowski, Zacharski, and Beck 1986), a clinical setting in which hemoglobin infusions might find use.

8.14 Synergism with Infection

In hemorrhagic shock in animals and humans, bacteria and endotoxin appear rapidly in the blood and may contribute to mortality (Rush et al. 1989). It is well known that the coincidence of blood and bacteria in a wound may be a life-threatening combination (Halsted 1891). Eaton, Brandt, and Mahoney (1982) found that the intraperitoneal administration of hemoglobin and bacteria in rats was much more lethal than either alone. Hemoglobin did not inhibit phagocytosis or neutrophil migration but Eaton and co-workers speculated that the bacteria were able to utilize hemoglobin iron. The addition of haptoglobin, which binds hemoglobin $\alpha\beta$ dimer, inhibited the hemoglobin effect. These authors concluded that haptoglobin may be an important natural defense in infection because it binds hemoglobin. Haptoglobin types 2–1 and 2–2 apparently also participate in the agglutination of some strains of *Streptococcus* (Kohler and Prokop 1978). Thus, completely saturating haptoglobin in large-volume hemoglobin resuscitations may be dangerous, particularly if bacteria are present.

The exact mechanism of binding of hemoglobin and haptoglobin is still not completely understood, but the carbohydrate groups on haptoglobin are important (Kaartinen and Monnen 1988). This raises the possibility that hemoglobin, free in solution, could bind to other molecules that contain glycoproteins such as bacterial cell walls.

8.15 Endotoxin

Endotoxin, whether bacterial or environmental, can cause agonizing problems in the production of hemoglobin solutions. Not only can endotoxin contaminate these solutions but they can cause biologic toxicities that can be confused with those attributed to hemoglobin itself. In particular, endotoxin has been shown to cause pulmonary hypertension (Hales et al. 1981), stimulation of myocytes (Shepherd, McDonough, and Burns 1986), and other cardiac dysfunction (Fish et al. 1985; Romanosky et al. 1986), but when perfused directly into the rat heart, it probably does not cause vasoconstriction (Artman et al. 1986). White, Murray, Smith et al. (1986) have suggested that hemoglobin and endotoxin may bind with a degree of specificity, and Chang (1990) suggested that endotoxin may contribute to mortality when hemoglobin is given to animals.

Studies on the infusion of purified bacterial endotoxins into humans (Suffredini et al. 1989) have shown that these substances can cause a flu-like syndrome and a hyperdynamic state, much like some of the side effects noted for hemoglobin solutions (see Chapter 10). Both pentoxifylline and ibuprofen seem to block the hyperdynamic state. It is possible that "environmental" endotoxins may have different biologic effects.

It is of interest that the lipopolysaccharide of endotoxin bears a resemblance to phospholipids found on the inner membrane of the red blood cell (Simoni et al. 1990). Perhaps this explains the toxicity noted for certain red blood cell membrane components and the observations that the method of lysis of red cells is crucial to limiting the toxicity of hemoglobin solutions.

The Food and Drug Administration has set a threshold of endotoxin contamination which produces pyrogen reaction in rabbits at 5.0 EU/kg or 1 ng/kg standard *Escherichia coli* endotoxin (Weary 1990). In a 70-kg man, this would correspond to a total dose of 350 EU. For a 4-unit transfusion (4 x 450 ml or 1,800 ml) this would mean that contamination with endotoxin could be no higher than 350/1,800 or about 0.25 EU/ml.

An additional problem with endotoxin is the possibility that hemoglobin either interferes with the assay or stimulates gelation of amoeba lysate. Cooper (1990) pointed out that the limulus amebocyte assay for endotoxin can be biased by suboptimal pH, endotoxin aggregation or adsorption, container effects, unbalanced cation concentrations, enzyme or protein modification, and nonspecific limulus amebocyte lysate activation. He recommended that about 90 percent of the problems can be overcome by dilution of the test materials since most problems are inhibition and concentration dependent.

Chapter 9

The Evaluation of Products

One of the largest problems caused by the commercialization of red cell substitutes is that products are not available for testing by impartial investigators. The Food and Drug Administration has not yet developed a set of evaluation procedures, and manufacturers provide little scientific information about their products, to protect patents and licenses and to avoid adverse publicity. Many of these manufacturers are relatively new small businesses and must be able to attract venture capital in order to survive. Publicity, whether in the lay press or peer-reviewed literature, may affect these businesses adversely.

Yet there is a real need to evaluate products according to scientifically accepted procedures so the products can be compared and and their safety established. At this time, there is no agreed-on set of evaluation procedures, and such a list is unlikely to be established because some tests cast products in good light, some in bad. Moreover, some products have known properties that may dictate special sets of studies.

Even though no commercial products are available at this time several classes of materials are under development (Table 9.1). In this

Table 9.1. Hemoglobin-based Products under Development

Pyridoxylated, polymerized hemoglobin (PLP-polyHb) (human, cow)
Cross-linked hemoglobin
Conjugated hemoglobin (polyethylene glycol, dextran)
Coascervates
Synthetic oxygen carriers (heme)
Encapsulated hemoglobin
Recombinant hemoglobin (bacteria, yeast, transgenic mammals)

chapter we will outline the procedures adopted at the Letterman Army Institute of Research to evaluate any product, whether of our own manufacture or from a commercial source (Table 9.2). The presentation is not exhaustive. Some preparations are tested in special ways or with special animal models to suit their special properties; thus detailed protocols are not given in this chapter.

Table 9.2. Evaluation Procedures for Hemoglobin-based Products

Oxygen transport
Oxygen capacity
Oxygen affinity (P_{50}, n, Bohr, CO_2 effects)
Purity and physical properties
Optical spectrum
Components: met-, CO, oxy-, deoxy-, sulf- hemoglobins
Electrolytes, pH, trace metals, lipids, phosphate
Endotoxin
HPLC: anion, cation, reversed phase
Electrophoresis, isoelectric focusing
Colloid osmotic pressure
Viscosity
Storage stability
Various temperatures, methemoglobin, spectrum, P_{50}, HPLC
Toxicity
Rabbit pyrogen test
Acute toxicity, rats
Serial killing, rats
Species differences: rat, rabbit, dog, pig, primate
Arterial vasoconstriction
Clinical trial simulation, primates
Endotoxin, bacterial clearance
Efficacy
O_2 transport
Clinical simulation (shock-resuscitation)
Biologic half-life
Metabolism
Immunogenicity

9.1 Oxygen Binding

The oxygen capacity of a solution cannot be equated to hemoglobin concentration because some derivatives of hemoglobin, such as methemoglobin, carboxyhemoglobin, or sulfhemoglobin, for example, bind no oxygen at all. Therefore, a direct method of measuring oxygen binding is necessary. This can be done with the older VanSlyke apparatus or with a newer technique such as the fuel cell, which measures oxygen liberated from oxyhemoglobin.

The oxygen equilibrium curve must be measured. Several techniques are available, but none of them is completely satisfactory. The older method of equilibrating samples with known mixtures of oxygen and measuring saturation with the VanSlyke or fuel cell is entirely satisfactory but cumbersome. Newer procedures using optical measurements of hemoglobin saturation are not acceptable because they depend on accurate knowledge of the absorption spectrum of the modified hemoglobin as well as assumptions about the fully saturated and unsaturated conditions. Systematic errors occur when the curve is progressively right-shifted (lower oxygen affinity). It is far better to have two or three accurate points on the curve than a continuous curve that is incorrect. Any measurement of P_{50} should be made under physiologic conditions (pH 7.4, PCO_2 40 torr, 37°C).

In addition to P_{50}, the degree of cooperativity, Hill's parameter (n), should be measured. This requires at least several points on the oxygen equilibrium curve around P_{50}, a few above and a few below. Hill's parameter should be expressed as its value at P_{50} since the actual value is saturation dependent.

The Bohr effect should be measured. This requires measuring P_{50} over a range of pH from about 7.0 to 7.8 (at constant PCO_2), with enough points so that a regression of log P_{50} versus pH can be established. The pH Bohr effect is expressed as the slope of this line. The carbon dioxide effect should be quantitated by measuring P_{50} at different carbon dioxide tensions but constant pH. In practice this can be very tedious since pH and PCO_2 are interdependent. These two Bohr effects should be measured with the product mixed with plasma to simulate in vivo conditions.

9.2 Purity and Physical Properties

An optical spectrum is mandatory. This should be measured between 450 and 650 nm using a spectrophotometer whose calibration can be established and traced to some reference standard. Some of the commercial instruments are not of sufficient quality to allow analysis of the optical spectrum.

Methemoglobin concentration is measured by any number of techniques, many depending on published extinction coefficients; thus they are only as good as the calibration of the spectrophotometer used for the measurements. Far better is the Evelyn-Malloy method, which is reproducible from laboratory to laboratory. Still better are the newer multicomponent methods, especially if each laboratory measures its own reference spectra for oxy-, deoxy-, met-, and carboxyhemoglobins.

Analysis of electrolytes, trace metals, lipids, and total phosphate must be carried out using standard reference methods. pH should be measured with an instrument whose calibration can be traced to standards of good quality. Careful attention should be paid to the temperature of calibration and measurement; they should both be 37°C.

Measurement of endotoxin is particularly important. Although newer chromogenic methods are now available, still the standard is the limulus amebocyte lysate assay (LAL). At the time of this writing, it is still not clear whether or not hemoglobin interferes with the LAL measurement. Therefore it is still impossible to specify whether one of the new automated techniques is satisfactory. In any case, it is imperative that if a low or negligible endotoxin measurement is made the solution be "spiked" with a known endotoxin reference sample to verify that the product does not interfere with the measurement.

High-pressure liquid chromatography (HPLC) is a rapidly advancing technique that is replacing conventional column methods. In general, anion, cation, and reversed phase columns are available, and all three should be used. These measurements should be accompanied by gel electrophoresis and isoelectric focusing.

Colloid osmotic pressure should be measured using an instrument specially designed for this purpose. Viscosity should be measured using a rotating (cone and plate) viscometer under a range of shear rates. The red cell substitute should be mixed with plasma and red cells under conditions likely to be encountered in clinical use (e.g., 50 percent hemodilution), and should be compared with whole blood at equivalent hemoglobin concentration.

9.3 Storage Stability

Stability under anticipated storage conditions should be studied, but measurement under conditions that can be reproduced in different laboratories should also be measured. Such studies should include, at the least, storage at ambient temperature (20°C), 4°C, -20°C, and -80°C. Vials should be prepared so they need not be entered repeatedly. Assay of stability should include an optical spectrum (above), methemoglobin concentration, and P_{50} determination. HPLC should be performed to evaluate possible degradation of components. Certain products may require additional testing depending on the type of instability anticipated.

Thermal stability is of interest and can be measured using a scanning calorimeter or simply by heating in a spectrophotometer cuvette that is thermostatted. Molecular weight distribution should be evaluated with those products that are polymerized or conjugated to higher molecular weight materials. It is particularly important to estimate the amount of uncross-linked hemoglobin in the preparation. Accumulation of aggregated material should be evaluated by filtration through a submicron filter. Gel electrophoresis and isoelectric focusing can also be helpful.

9.4 Toxicity

As demonstrated by the earlier discussion of hemoglobin toxicity, many facets of the effects of hemoglobin in vivo need to be evaluated in order to establish safety. It must be recognized that any organ or organ system is at risk of toxicity, and so an organized survey must be undertaken. In addition, hemoglobin and/or its contaminants, either from red cell stroma or the manufacturing process, may be responsible for toxicity. Furthermore, components of hemoglobin, $\alpha\beta$ dimers, heme, methemoglobin, or hemichromes may contribute additional toxicity.

Different protocols need to be tailored for each product and designed to evaluate particular properties of the solutions. But certain tests should be standard so that solutions can be compared.

9.4.1 Rabbit Pyrogen Test

A single injection, calculated to be 20 percent of the total blood volume, should be given by ear vein. Monitoring should include electrocardiogram, temperature and blood pressure. Five animals should be studied because of the variation in responsiveness to this test. White blood cell and platelet counts should be followed in the hour after administration.

9.4.2 Acute Toxicity

Rats should be used for this test even though they are extremely resistant to the toxic effects of hemoglobin. An 80 percent blood volume exchange should be carried out by tail vein. Survival after 24 hours should be noted, and all animals should be killed to study histology with special attention to the liver, kidneys, and eyes.

9.4.3 Serial Killing

In a separate set of studies, a similar 80 percent exchange transfusion should be carried out, but the animals should be killed at intervals to study the time course of lesions noted in the acute toxicity studies above.

9.4.4 Species Variation

Differences in reactivity in different species should be studied by injections of bolus amounts into several species including rats, rabbits, pigs, primates, and dogs. A dose of 20 percent of estimated blood volume is standard, and the same study can be used to evaluate the plasma retention half-time. Not only survival but temperature, electrocardiogram, and blood pressure should be followed.

9.4.5 Vasoconstriction

Arterial vasoconstriction should be measured in a physiologic model such as the isolated, perfused rabbit heart (Langendorf preparation). The hearts should be perfused first with oxygenated Krebs-Henseleit buffer, and then with the test solution in concentrations up to about 2 g/dl. Increases in the left ventricular developed pressure should be monitored. After a steady state is achieved with the hemoglobin solution, the perfusion should be switched back to buffer, and baseline should be reestablished before retesting the hemoglobin at a different dose. The relationship between hemoglobin concentration and pressure change should be established.

9.4.6 Renal Toxicity

Renal function tests should receive special attention. These should include creatinine clearance, quantitation of sodium reabsorption, urine concentration (specific gravity), and microscopic examination for sediment and cells. The hemoglobin content of urine should be measured, and if appreciable amounts appear, the samples should be concentrated and identification of the hemoglobin species should be carried out using HPLC or electrophoretic analysis.

In addition to renal function tests, careful histologic examination of necropsy specimens should be done because in many cases in which abnormal function is not detected histologic changes do occur. When demonstrated, the time course of recovery from such damage should be documented.

9.4.7 Clinical Trial Simulation in Primates

Since the Savitsky study showed certain toxic effects in humans it should be carried out in primates before humans. A dose of 0.25 g/kg should be administered at about 2–3 ml/min. At the very minimum, urine output, blood pressure, and electrocardiogram should be monitored. In addition, helpful information would include the amount of hemoglobin cleared in the urine, creatinine clearance, and liver function tests. Reticulocytes should be counted daily along with complete blood counts. Blood smears should be made in anticipation of changes in red cells, white cells, or platelets which can be supported by morphologic examination. Coagulation, prothrombin time, and partial thromboplastin times should be followed daily along with complement activation.

9.4.8 Endotoxin, Bacterial Clearance

The tendency for the red cell substitute to contribute to bacterial growth or to inhibit the clearance of bacteria should be evaluated by suitable studies of infusion of bacteria or injury to the gut.

9.5 Efficacy

Efficacy is perhaps the most difficult property of red cell substitute solutions to establish. Two objectives should be sought: demonstration of oxygen transport and simulation of an anticipated clinical usage. The first is the most straightforward and can be carried out by demonstrating survival in the absence of red cells in any of a number of animals.

Oxygen transport can be established using the isolated, perfused heart model described above. Alternatively, animals can be completely exchange transfused with the candidate solution to hematocrits that are known to be lethal. This is not a clinically relevant procedure because the solutions will never be used in this way; rather, this protocol is designed to establish that the solutions do carry oxygen under in vivo conditions.

The second objective, clinical simulation, is much more difficult because it requires the anticipation of clinical application. In the case of shock resuscitation, a model must be developed first. For example, controlled hemorrhage to a predetermined blood pressure can be carried out, and the animal can be kept in the shock state for a time. Then resuscitation can be carried out using the blood substitute candidate. Controls should always include albumin (protein, colloid effects), Ringer's lactate, and whole blood. The animal chosen for this study could be pig or primate; the rat is so resistant to physiologic damage from hemorrhage that its usefulness is questionable.

9.6 Biologic Half-life

The biologic (plasma) half-life is dependent on the dose and species studied; therefore it is important to explore both of these variables. In humans the plasma retention will not be known until human trials are performed. Twenty and 50 percent blood volume infusions should be done in rat, rabbit, pig, and monkey. In at least one of these species a broader range of concentrations should be given to establish a detailed analysis of the dose dependence.

9.7 Metabolism

The metabolic pattern of the proposed red cell substitute should be established. The reagent used to modify hemoglobin should be labeled radioactively so that its disappearance from key organs, including brain, heart, liver, and kidneys, can be followed, as well as its presence in urine and feces. Of interest would be the fate of different parts of the hemoglobin molecule, including heme, protein, and iron.

9.8 Immunogenicity

It is essential to establish immunogenicity of red cell substitutes so that a policy regarding repeated usage can be established. Unfortunately, there are no accepted methods for quantitating immunogenicity since hemoglobin is generally not a good antigen. However, a model could be established which includes repeated immunization with the test materials to animals such as rabbits. Specific antibodies to the modified hemoglobin must be sought over time, and a relationship between the degree of antigenicity and degree of modification must be established. In addition to the formation of antibodies, activation of the broader immune system should be evaluated. Thus, studies of basophil activation (histamine release), coagulation cascades, platelet activation, and prostaglandin synthesis would be of interest. Interleukins, tumor necrosis factor, and thromboxane generation should be studied.

9.9 Microcirculation

Many of the known toxic effects of hemoglobin solutions might be explained on the basis of their interactions with the endothelium. Therefore, we have undertaken studies of the biologic interactions of hemoglobin with cultured endothelial cells. In addition, there are a number of specialized laboratories that can visualize directly the interactions of red blood cells, leukocytes, and platelets with the vascular endothelium. These techniques should provide valuable correlations with the hemoglobin-cell interaction studies discussed above.

9.10 "Stress" Models

Past experience with clinical trials has suggested that normal volunteers and patients may react differently to massive infusions of hemoglobin solutions. Although the reasons for this suspicion are not as yet understood, it is possible that patients have already activated cell-mediated immune (macrophage) systems, be depleted of haptoglobin or other heme-binding proteins, or have bacteremia or endotoxemia. Thus is it important in preclinical trials to study not only normal, healthy animals, but also models of surgical stress, trauma, infection, or compromised immunity. Many specific protocols are available.

In our institute, standardized shock models are available. Animals are hemorrhaged to a predetermined blood pressure, held there for a time, then resuscitated with the test solution. Because hemoglobin is known to support bacterial growth we believe infection is also a good model for study.

9.11 Clinical Models

The clinical application for which the candidate red cell substitute is intended should dictate some of the specific efficacy and safety studies to be carried out in the preclinical phase of development.

Perhaps the most demanding of these clinical settings is resuscitation from blood loss because of the complexity of interactions among ischemia, hypotension, hypoxia, infection, and endotoxemia. It should be remembered that in most trauma therapy, not only are resuscitation solutions given, but all patients eventually receive blood, saline, and coagulation factors. Thus, to evaluate the potential usefulness of a resuscitation solution, a protocol should be designed in which the insult is followed by treatment only with the candidate solution to simulate its field use. After a period of time the animal should have available to it all of the resources of the modern intensive care unit and other intravenous solutions if that is the anticipated clinical use.

Development of applications such as angioplasty, intraoperative hemodilution, or hypothermia would require other protocols for preclinical evaluation. Perhaps many of these would be much less demanding than shock-resuscitation.

These studies are intended only to be guidelines and reflect procedures now used in our institition. The studies are very expensive, especially the tests using animals. But the important point to be made is that a "core" of protocols is being accepted de facto by workers in the field, and it would probably be extremely helpful to developers and evaluaters alike to adopt a common set of protocols so that products can be compared. In reviewing the literature it is very impressive that clinical trials that revealed toxic effects in humans had been used in animal tests without significant toxicity. Therefore, scrupulous standardization of safety testing is not only desirable but essential.

Chapter 10
Clinical Trials

The ultimate test of a blood substitute solution is infusion into human subjects. Because of early interest in the mechanism of transfusion reactions and consequent renal failure, a number of studies are available for examination. Many were done with only tracer amounts of hemoglobin and so do not represent therapeutic doses. But the studies provide data of interest in considering safety.

The published literature represents only a fraction of the human subjects who have received intravenous hemoglobin. Some studies have not been published because untoward reactions were observed, and other trials were carried out in foreign countries in which publication in the open literature is not encouraged.

Because many of the published studies were not done to evaluate hemoglobin as a blood substitute but to study its metabolism, some information is not available such as infusion rates, hemoglobin concentration, and plasma or urine concentrations. Some of the early studies paid little attention to a clinical evaluation of the recipients. In still others, the solutions used were not described in detail. Nevertheless, it is useful to glean what information we can from these reports, and it is the goal of this chapter to attempt to dissect the major toxicities seen in human subjects.

Who first administered hemoglobin solutions to humans for therapeutic purposes is difficult to determine. Sellards and Minot (1916) cite an earlier paper by Benczur (*Deutsch Arch f klin Med* 36:388, 1885) as the first. Apparently Sellards and Minot administered hemoglobin subcutaneously and observed local inflammation reactions. But the first to administer hemoglobin and report the experience in the modern literature was VonStark.

10.1 VonStark

VonStark (1898) administered hemoglobin subcutaneously into six anemic patients. The amount of hemoglobin was increased from 10 ml of a 0.25 g/dl solution to 5 ml of a 10 g/dl solution. These were tolerated well. Although there was a little swelling and local pain at the site of injection no other untoward effects were noted. VonStark was not able to prepare stable solutions that resisted decomposition and therefore terminated his studies.

10.2 Sellards and Minot

Sellards and Minot (1916) prepared hemoglobin solutions by washing human red cells and lysing them in distilled water. The final solutions were made isotonic with a concentrated salt solution. A total of thirty-three subjects received injections, ranging from 5 to 33 ml of solution containing 1–10 g of hemoglobin; sufficient material was given to induce hemoglobinuria. Of these subjects, thirty had no reportable ill effects. Three subjects experienced fever (two with chills), and one who received 33 ml of the hemoglobin solution had chills, headache, fever, nausea, flushing, and difficulty sleeping.

10.3 Ottenberg and Fox

Ottenberg and Fox (1938) reported on the injection of hemoglobin into twenty normal volunteers. The solution was prepared by washing pooled red cells with saline, lysing in water, and filtering through a Seitz filter. The doses ranged from 3.47 to 8.25 g over a period of five to twelve minutes. Little clinical information is given in their report, but the authors found "no untoward symptoms."

10.4 O'Shaughnessy, Mansell, and Slome

O'Shaughnessy, Mansell, and Slome (1939) infused hemoglobin solution into four cancer patients who had been alkalinized. The material had been prepared according to Amberson, Flexner, et al. (1934–35) and 10–50 g was administered over thirty to sixty minutes in a volume of 200–1,000 ml. The effects included flushing in one patient, dyspnea in one, chest "tightness" in two, lower back pain in two, "rigor" in three, and tachycardia in one.

10.5 Fairly

Fairly (1940) also prepared hemoglobin as a centrifuged water lysate of human red cells, 13.8 g/dl concentration, and infused it into three subjects. Two subjects who received 14 and 17 g of hemoglobin had no reaction. The third, who received 21 g, experienced nausea and fever.

10.6 Gilligan, Altschule, and Katersky

Gilligan and co-workers (1941) again prepared a water lysate of human red cells and centrifuged it to remove stroma. Fifteen injections were given to ten volunteers. Two who received 10–16 g of hemoglobin had abdominal cramps and vomiting for forty minutes after the injections. One who received 16 g had chills preceding the onset of abdominal pain.

10.7 Cannan and Redish

Cannan and Redish (1942) also prepared a water lysate of human red cells and centrifuged it. Test doses were given to dogs before infusion into human volunteers. Fever and chills were noted in the subject who received 0.33 g/kg, ninety minutes after the infusion; the temperature was normal in one hour. At the highest dose given, 0.64 g/kg, one subject developed nausea, fever, and abdominal pain that lasted five hours, and a second subject had nausea, vomiting, and abdominal pain, but no fever. In contrast, a subject who received 0.7 g/kg, had no untoward effects.

10.8 Amberson, Jennings, and Rhode

Amberson, Jennings, and Rhode (1949) reported 77 infusions of hemoglobin-Ringer's in fourteen patients. The hemoglobin solution was prepared by toluene lysis of human red cells and filtering to remove stroma. They observed a rise in blood pressure and fall in pulse rate even when the volumes of hemoglobin were too small to affect blood volume. Oliguria occurred in one patient, three had rises in blood urea nitrogen (BUN) and decreased urea clearance, and in one there was a drop in glomerular filtration rate. Amberson and his co-workers focused most of their attention on one patient, a woman who suffered from postpartum hemorrhage. She was given multiple infusions of hemoglobin solutions, totaling 2,300 ml. Despite stabilization of the hemodynamics, the patient's oliguria worsened, and she died in renal failure. Amberson felt that this case showed both the potential of hemoglobin solutions (cardiovascular stabilization) and their danger (renal failure), and he concluded that a safe solution had not yet been found.

10.9 Brandt, Frank, and Lichtman

Brandt and his colleagues (1951) prepared hemoglobin solutions according to a slightly different method. They administered their solutions to eight patients who had no evidence of renal disease and to six with the nephrotic syndrome. Both groups showed a reduced urine flow, renal plasma flow (mean reduction, 41 percent), and glomerular filtration rate. Brandt and his co-workers concluded that because of nephrotoxicity hemoglobin solutions should not be used when the patient is in shock or in any situation in which renal function is impaired.

10.10 Miller and McDonald

Miller and McDonald (1951) performed similar infusions of hemoglobin solution in twenty-six normal human volunteers. Their solutions were prepared by the method of Pennell and Smith (1949). They noted (1) an increase in diastolic and systolic blood pressures; (2) a decrease in pulse rate; (3) a decrease in the clearance of inulin and paraamino hippuric acid; (4) an increase in filtration fraction; (5) a decrease in urine flow; and (6) an increase in the percent of the glomerular filtrate reabsorbed by the renal tubules. They believed that these effects were caused by renal vasoconstriction and that this was a property of cell-free hemoglobin.

10.11 Phillips and Coworkers

Phillips et al. (1951) reported on a navy project that studied the infusion of hemoglobin solutions into humans. Two types of solution were developed by Merck, Sharp, and Dohme: one, a liquid, was prepared according to Hamilton and co-workers and the other, lyophilized, was by the procedure of Pennell and Smith (1949). The subjects of the study were patients hospitalized in Egypt for louse-borne relapsing fever with anemia. Urea clearance, heart rate, blood pressure, respiratory rate, and rectal temperature were measured. Forty-seven patients received sixty-two infusions of 6–7 g/dl hemoglobin solution at rates between 30 and 50 ml/minute.

Thirty-five of the subjects had no temperature elevation. In the other seventeen, the heart rate dropped immediately after the infusions, and the blood pressure rose. Urea clearance dropped immediately. The authors had the impression that hemoglobin solutions that had been stored for prolonged periods or that had been frozen and rethawed were more likely to cause problems. One patient who received a solution that had been thawed and refrozen at least twice developed oliguria and an elevated BUN. This patient's BUN and urea clearance returned to normal by the follow-up examination three years later. No renal impairment was noted in forty out of fifty-two infusions with frozen hemoglobin, but twenty of these forty had other side effects; it was therefore concluded that the presence of untoward effects or symptoms was not a guide to renal involvement.

Ten patients were followed up three years after the protocol studies. Two had severe renal damage, three had mild damage, and five had no renal dysfunction. At retesting, none of these patients had demonstrable renal compromise.

In a separate study, the authors reconstituted lyophilized hemoglobin that had been stored for two years at $4^{0}C$. The solution was 6–7 g/dl and was given to one patient at a rate of 100 ml/minute. Phillips and colleagues observed no evidence of renal failure as judged by BUN or creatinine clearance. One patient had a "typical infusion reaction" that was attributed to breakdown of the rubber in the infusion set.

10.12 Lathem

Lathem (1959) studied the renal clearance of hemoglobin by administering a hemoglobin solution to ten normal volunteers. The amount of total hemoglobin given was 14–18 g over four hours. Lathem noted that the renal threshold for hemoglobin appears to be 128 mg/dl, but no clinical observations were included. Presumably there were no ill effects.

10.13 Garby and Noyes

Garby and Noyes (1959) reported the kinetics of the disappearance of hemoglobin from the circulation. The hemolysate, prepared from a subject with polycythemia vera, was produced by freezing and thawing and filtering through a Seitz filter. The final concentration was 22–38 mg/ml. Infusions were done in twelve normal volunteers, and no ill effects were noted.

10.14 Spector and Crosby

Spector and Crosby (1975) carried out a study of infusion of lysed red cells to try to determine if abnormalities of coagulation would result.

They collected 100–150 ml of autologous blood from healthy volunteers and prepared lysates by freezing and thawing. In ten subjects, 100 ml of solution was injected over a ten-minute period. Four received 50 ml over a three- to four- minute period, and then a continuous infusion over five hours was carried out to maintain plasma hemoglobin at about 250 mg/dl. These authors reported that all infusions were asymptomatic. Although no significant coagulation defects were noted the platelets dropped within five minutes after the beginning of the infusions but were normal by 30 minutes. No evidence for disseminated intravascular coagulation was found.

10.15 Rabiner

In a symposium held at the National Institutes of Health in 1974, Rabiner (1975) reported on the use of hemoglobin solutions in trauma cases in the Soviet Union. He stated that the method being used there produced a solution of 3 g/dl hemoglobin which was heavily contaminated with stromal lipid. Specifically, thirty patients received 200–400 ml of hemoglobin with "stabilization of blood pressure and overall clinical benefit."

One separate Soviet scientist administered 14–15 ml/kg hemoglobin to sixteen patients, and one was given 2 liters. These patients had marked hematuria, a plasma hemoglobin concentration of 0.5–0.7 g/dl, and a 50 percent loss over four hours. Creatinine and urea clearances were said to be normal. Rabiner concluded his remarks by stating, "One of our pharmaceutical companies is working on developing a stroma-free hemoglobin solution. . . . I am hopeful that in the near future, a preparation of hemoglobin solution will be available for clinical trials" (p. 1457).

10.16 Savitsky and Coworkers

Encouraged by the reports of Rabiner and others on the positive effect of hemoglobin purification, Savitsky et al. (1978) carried out a study of "Rabiner" hemoglobin in human volunteers. The hemoglobin solutions used in this study were prepared by the Warner-Lambert Company (Table 10.1). It was prepared from outdated human blood, lysed by hypotonic phosphate buffer, and filtered through a 0.22 micron filter. It was dialyzed against $NaHCO_3$, and salts were adjusted to the concentrations shown in Table 10.1.

Preliminary studies in animals were done to test the solutions. Prior tests in animals by Peskin, O'Brien and Rabiner (1968) and by Relihan and Litwin (1972, 1973) had shown no ill effects in normal dogs or in dogs with renal ischemia or acidosis. Birndorf and Lopas (1969) had also shown no adverse effects of similar solutions in monkeys, and Savitsky stated that they had tested the solutions in dogs and monkeys further prior to use in the human studies. Exchange transfusions were carried out in dogs to hematocrits between 1 and 10 percent. All survived acutely, and the hemoglobin solutions were found to transport O_2. Savitsky felt that as a plasma expander after acute hemorrhage the solution was superior to dextran 70 or 5 percent albumin.

Table 10.1. Hemoglobin Solution Used by Savitsky and Co-workers.

Analysis	Result
Calcium	4.5 mEq/liter
Magnesium	1.9 mEq/liter
Potassium	4.0 mEq/liter
Sodium	140.0 mEq/liter
Chloride	98.0 mEq/liter
Hemoglobin	6.4 g/dl
Methemoglobin	1.2 % of total
pH	7.09
Lipid phosphorus	0.02 mg/dl
Coagulant activity	negative
Pyrogen test	negative
LD_{50}	>100 ml/kg
Sterility	passed
Hepatitis B surface antigen	negative

Source: data from Savitsky et al. (1978).

The human subjects for the study were eight normal volunteers. The hemoglobin solutions, 0.25 g/kg, were infused at a rate of 2 ml/min in two subjects and at 4 ml/min in another six. Two of the patients who received the faster infusion rate developed abdominal and bilateral costovertebral angle pain. Seven of the eight volunteers developed bradycardia

(Fig. 10.1) and a rise in blood pressure, and all showed transient oliguria and fall in creatinine clearance. The peak urine hemoglobin concentration was 10–57 mg/dl, and the peak serum hemoglobin concentration was 57 mg/dl (average), with a range 13–100 mg/dl.

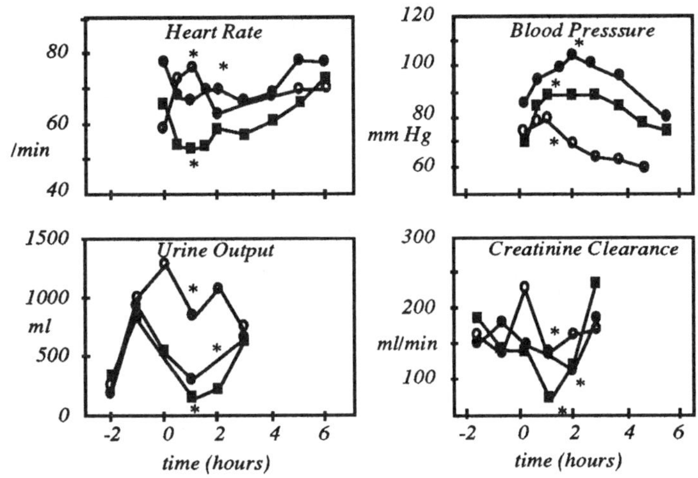

Figure 10.1. Changes in heart rate, blood pressure, urine output, and creatinine clearance after infusion of hemoglobin solution to human volunteers. *Solid circles*, 2 ml/min. *Solid squares*, 4 ml/min. *Open circles*, albumin control, 4 ml/min. * marks end of infusions. Hemoglobin infusions caused a dose-dependent drop in heart rate, rise in blood pressure, and decreased urine output. *Source:* data from Savitsky et al. (1978).

Savitsky and his colleagues concluded that the drop in urine flow and creatinine clearance was caused by a drop in renal plasma flow, probably by vasoconstriction. They believed this effect was probably due to hemoglobin itself, not stroma, because the solutions were "stroma-free." They had no explanation for bradycardia but noted the earlier work of Miller and McDonald (1951), who had demonstrated similar findings.

10.17 Moss and Coworkers

Moss et al. reported the first clinical trial of modified hemoglobin in humans (Table 10.2). The solution used was pyridoxylated hemoglobin, polymerized with glutaraldehyde (PLP-polyHb). Six healthy volunteers were hydrated with intravenous Ringer's lactate and oral water, and then hemoglobin solution, 0.25 g/kg, was infused. Five of the subjects tolerated the procedure well, whereas the sixth had a "mild allergic response." The peak plasma hemoglobin level was 432 ± 23 mg/dl. These authors concluded that their results did not show renal toxicity or coagulation defects and that polyhemoglobin is safe for further human trials.

Table 10.2. Renal Function after Infusion of PLP-polyHb

	Pre-infusion	Post-infusion	p
Creatinine Clearance (ml/min)	113 ± 11	119 ± 3	NS[a]
Urine flow (ml/min)	7.7 ± 1.2	6.3 ± 0.4	NS
Urine osm (mosm/kg)	178 ± 13	179 ± 22	NS
Urine Na^+ (mEq/liter)	59 ± 4.0	57 ± 9	NS

Source: data from Moss et al. (1989).
Note: Values are mean ± S.E.
[a] NS, not significant.

10.18 Summary of Human Trials

In all, seventeen studies in more than 211 human subjects have been published. At this time, an additional five studies of the infusion of modified hemoglobin into humans have been carried out, but all are still unpublished. Only one study of modified hemoglobin has been published and that only as a meeting abstract (Moss et al. 1989). Amberson reported the death of one patient in hemorrhagic shock who received hemoglobin solution as a last resort; this patient had renal failure at the time of death.

Table 10.3. Summary of Side Effects in Clinical Trials

Side Effect	Frequency
Renal	
Oliguria	24/36
Decreased renal plasma flow	40/40
Increased BUN	3/14
Decreased GFR	14/14
Decreased creatinine clearance	9/22
WBC in sediment	3/8
System	
Death	1/211 (shock)
Fever	2/36
Chills	3/43
Nausea	2/36
Headache	1/33
Flushing	2/37
Vomiting	2/10
"Allergic"	1/6
Cardiovascular	
Tachycardia	1/4
Bradycardia	50/81
Hypertension	26/55
Other	
Rigor	3/4
Lower back pain	2/4
CVA tenderness	1/8
Chest pain	2/4
Dyspnea	1/4
Abdominal	5/28
Hematologic	
Decreased platelets	10/10 (hemolysate)
Increased PTT	8/8

Note: The abbreviations used are: BUN, blood urea nitrogen; GFR, glomerular filtration rate; WBC, white blood cell count; PTT, partial thromboplastin time; CVA, costovertebral angle.

Table 10.3 summarizes the accumulated side effects of hemoglobin-based red cell substitutes. The data in this table cannot be regarded as exact because the studies span ninety-one years, and methods of reporting, methods used, and emphasis have changed. In some of the studies, notably those designed to follow the metabolism and excretion of hemoglobin, little mention is made of the clinical consequences of the infusions, and in some no measurements of vital signs or blood values were made. Nevertheless, it is striking that at least 89 of the 211 total subjects had no ill effects.

Most prominent among the untoward effects are those involving the kidney. Oliguria is a very frequent finding, and when observed, renal plasma flow is almost always reduced. The study of Savitsky et al. (1978) found oliguria and decreased creatinine clearance in eight of eight subjects studied. The more recent work of the Moss group used a modified hemoglobin that is not cleared by the kidney, supporting their hypothesis that if renal clearance can be prevented, oliguria will not occur. It should be emphasized that the nature of the renal effect is not known. Vasoconstriction and tubular obstruction have been suggested, but tubule cell damage by reabsorbed hemoglobin might also occur. In addition, increased colloid osmotic pressure by unpolymerized hemoglobin would be expected to reduce the oncotic force contributing to glomerular filtration.

Although most concern has been with renal toxicity, other effects are also prominent. Bradycardia and hypertension are frequent findings. No explanation for these effects has been advanced, and it is disturbing that no animal model for study seems to have been developed. Moreover, bradycardia and systemic hypertension are not features of hemolytic transfusion reaction, suggesting a different mechanism.

Systemic reactions such as fever and chills are rare, but flushing, nausea, and chest and abdominal pain are prominent. A dose dependence is difficult to establish for these effects.

Chapter 11
Summary and Conclusions

11.1 History

A brief examination of the history of transfusion therapy shows clearly that red cell substitutes have been sought since the concept of the circulation of the blood was first discovered in the seventeenth century. Initially, substitutes were desired as alternatives to transfusion of homologous (same species) or heterologous (other species) blood because of known dangers of those procedures.

Perhaps the most important point brought out in this historical examination is that transfusions were not safe until advances occurred in allied areas of science. These advances included an understanding of the coagulation mechanism, bacterial contamination, and blood groups. So it is with any transition of scientific concepts to applications in human use: if there are major gaps in our collective knowledge in areas crucial to development of the product then efforts are doomed regardless of the effort invested. The central issue in the development of a safe substitute for red cells is whether or not we now possess knowledge of all the biologic mechanisms needed to produce a safe product.

In the past the needs that have stimulated the search for a red cell substitute have been largely military. The military is the only guaranteed customer for products, and much scientific work was done in and after World War II. Since the end of World War II, the U.S. military has continued to support research and development of products for use on the battlefield.

In recent years a major new stimulus, AIDS, has carried the attractiveness of these products out of the military and into civilian circles, with the resultant influx of venture capital and new pressures on scientists to strive to meet deadlines in their research. A danger is that these new forces will drive product development around the usual hurdles of proper peer review and publication in the open literature.

11.2 Clinical Indications

Red cell transfusion in the United States is big business and is not likely to diminish, regardless of progress in red cell substitutes. In fact, it is speculated that if such materials are available and if they are safe, transfusions will increase, not decrease; but newer, aggressive medical therapies that require large amounts of blood, such as liver transplantation and other procedures, will be developed.

In the nineteenth century, one of the leading indications for transfusion therapy was thought to be resurrection: infusion into corpses to restore life. This is interesting because when transfusion became possible many other applications were developed, and even this initial one proved to be ridiculous. So it is with red cell substitutes. It is very likely that initial applications will be for resuscitation, hemodilution, and so on; but when products are available, their unique properties will suggest applications not imagined now.

Other applications that are anticipated now include reperfusion of ischemic tissue such as myocardium after infarction, extracorporeal organ perfusion for storage, cell culture media, and for cardioplegia, hematopoietic stimulation, sickle-cell anemia, tumor therapy, and chronic anemia. It must be emphasized that research uses will be extremely important. The new products will allow investigation into basic mechanisms of oxygen transport and tissue oxygenation which have been impossible up to now.

Some of the required specifications for a red cell substitute are obvious: sterility, long shelf life, and so on. But their physiologic properties are not so clear-cut. The P_{50} should not be lower than about 19 torr, but the upper limit is not as easy to determine. This is because whether or not a hemoglobin with high P_{50} can transport oxygen to tissues effectively depends on whether or not it is fully saturated on the arterial side of the circulation.

The capacity to carry oxygen is also not known exactly, but to use a rule of thumb, the objective of therapy should be to keep the patient's hemoglobin concentration above 8–10 g/dl. The balance between oxygen capacity and flow properties is complex.

The viscosity of the solution should be the lowest achievable. Such solutions will be advantageous in the perfusion of ischemic tissues, infusion through catheter lumens that are being used increasingly by all sorts of machinery, and to open up capillary beds constricted by shock. Special attention should be paid to mixtures of red cell substitutes and red cells in proportions likely to be encountered in clinical practice.

The desired plasma retention time is also not known exactly. Certainly persistence for more than a few hours is attractive, but is a plasma half-life of several days really necessary? This question is important in regard to modification because in order to achieve long retention times hemoglobin molecules must be either polymerized or conjugated to other polymers. Both of these steps introduce additional potential toxicity problems. The answer to this question will likely await introduction of the first generation of clinical products so that some experience in their use can be gained.

The optimal colloid osmotic pressure will depend on the clinical application. Recent work in resuscitation solutions indicates that hyperoncotic solutions are very useful in hemorrhagic shock, and these solutions are attractive to the military who must reduce weight and cube to a minimum for logistical reasons. But in other clinical applications, isooncotic solutions with the highest possible oxygen capacity would be desired.

Physician acceptance is an interesting issue. How will physicians react to a choice between natural and synthetic products? They will probably be influenced more by the benefit/risk ratio, safety of handling, and ease of use than by cost. Thus, it is important to begin to consider how the products will be used in terms of adjunct monitoring and therapy such as fluids and electrolytes, colloid, and so on. Another issue is the difficulty or ease of teaching medical students, house officers, and technicians to use the new products.

It is not clear yet who will "control" the use of the new products. Will it be the blood bank, intensive care physicians, or pharmacists? So far, academic blood bankers have not been eager to step to the lead in the development of new products; rather, surgeons seem to have been the most active, with anesthesiologists and internists developing interest. Perhaps the National Red Cross will develop a policy in the near future in regard to the collection of blood for modification and distribution of eventual products. In any case, it is likely that red cell substitutes will change the way medicine is practiced.

The Federal Food, Drug, and Cosmetic Act (21 U.S.C. 360) classifies blood and blood products as drugs, and Section 351 of the Public Health Service Act (42 U.S.C. 262) classifies these products as biologic products. The first step in commercializing a product is for the manufacturer to demonstrate the product's safety and effectiveness when it is used according to the directions provided by the manufacturer and approved by the Food and Drug Administration (FDA).

The manufacturer must first file with the appropriate section of the

FDA a Notice of Claimed Investigational Exemption for a New Drug (IND). The purpose of this step is to protect human subjects from premature human use and to ensure that such volunteers or patients are adequately informed about the nature and risks of the clinical studies to be performed. During this process, the manufacturer presents data collected in animal studies which establish the product's safety. Once the IND application is approved, the manufacturer then sets about collecting data on the safety and efficacy of the product in humans.

According to the FDA, *safety* means "the relative freedom from harmful effect to persons affected, directly or indirectly, by a product when prudently administered, taking into consideration the character of the product in relation to the condition of the recipient at the time. Proof of safety shall consist of adequate tests by methods reasonably applicable to show the biological product is safe under the prescribed conditions of use, including significant human experience during use" (Barker 1975, 1523). *Efficacy* means "a reasonable expectation that, in a significant proportion of the target population, the pharmacologic or other effect of the biological product, when used under adequate directions for use and warnings against unsafe use, will serve a clinically significant function in the diagnosis, cure, mitigation, treatment, or prevention of disease in man. Proof of effectiveness shall consist of controlled clinical investigations" (Barker 1975, 1523).

When the appropriate data have been collected, the censure process starts. During this often prolonged procedure, the FDA reviews all data, generally consulting with experts in the scientific community to obtain the best advice before a decision is made. The granting of a license is based upon the manufacturers' compliance with good manufacturing practices and their adherence to published standards for products. Product standards are developed in consultation with the scientific community and are published in the *Federal Register* to allow a period for comments by the public. These standards are subject to change as knowledge about specific types of products accumulates.

In the area of hemoglobin-based red cell substitutes, there is no precedent at the FDA for licensing products. Therefore there are no published standards against which new products can be measured. Rigorous demonstration of efficacy for hemoglobin solutions still has not been demonstrated because satisfactory products have not been available for testing. Safety remains a major problem at this time because of the enormous literature on the toxicity of hemoglobin solutions. As discussed in Chapter 8, the consensus in the field is that toxicity of such solutions is caused by impurities, but definite proof is still lacking. Manufacturing standards cannot be established yet because the "impurities" or properties of hemoglobin solutions that have been toxic in the past are not yet defined completely. Clearly, the FDA must "feel its way" cautiously in regard to these important issues as it accumulates a body of information upon which to develop standards for these new products.

11.3 Structure and Function of Hemoglobin

Hemoglobin is probably the most studied and best understood human protein. It is composed of four subunit polypeptide chains, each one of which contains an iron-porphyrin group, heme, that can bind oxygen. When the concentration of hemoglobin is less than that found in the red cell, the molecule tends to dissociate into subunits, each with two smaller subunits. In this way, the body clears cell-free hemoglobin from the circulation since the dimers are readily filtered in the kidney.

There are major gaps in our understanding of the details of the function of hemoglobin. Its primary structure is known at the atomic level, and the integration of its structure is so delicate that a change of only one amino acid can lead to disastrous consequences, as demonstrated by point mutations such as sickle-cell anemia.

Tertiary and quaternary structures of hemoglobin give rise to its important physiologic properties: oxygen affinity suitable for tissue oxygenation, the Bohr (pH) effect, carbon dioxide effect, 2,3-diphosphoglycerate (2,3-DPG) effect, and cooperativity. Although these properties are present in all known hemoglobins in higher organisms, the exact necessity in biologic function is still unknown, and how critical these properties are in pathologic situations such as anemia or hypoxia is even less well understood.

The oxygen equilibrium curve (OEC) of hemoglobin is the standard way of relating the hemoglobin saturation to dissolved oxygen concentration, or tension (PO_2). Measurement of the OEC is one of the essential ways of evaluating the ability of a solution to transport oxygen. Cooperativity is expressed by the sigmoid (S) shape of the curve, and the overall oxygen affinity is expressed by its position (P_{50}, or PO_2 at half-saturation).

Chemical modifications of hemoglobin change its basic structure-function relationships, and the nature of these perturbations provides information not only about the physiologic effects of hemoglobin but also about the site and nature of the modification. Several theoretical models of hemoglobin oxygen binding have been described, but none is entirely satisfactory in explaining observed phenomena.

The most useful of the models describes the function of hemoglobin according to the "two-state" theory because it details two distinct structures, one corresponding to oxyhemoglobin and the other to deoxyhemoglobin. These two structures have essentially different affinities for oxygen: oxygen binds first to the low affinity, deoxy conformation, which, by virtue of binding oxygen, switches to a higher affinity form. This switch accounts for the cooperative nature of oxygen binding. All of the various chemical modifications proposed to produce red cell substitutes interfere in one way or another with this delicate balance between conformations and have some effect on cooperativity and oxygen affinity. The state of the art is not yet at the point that prediction of consequences can be made from knowledge of structural alterations although serious advances toward this goal have been achieved in recent years.

11.4 Physiology of Oxygen Transport

Higher organisms have a circulatory system because simple diffusion of oxygen from the environment to sites of mitochondrial respiration is impossible. Oxygen transport is thus the sum total of many different processes, including breathing, transfer of oxygen from the alveolar space to pulmonary capillary blood, reaction with hemoglobin, diffusion into and out of the red cell, and diffusion to tissue sites.

According to the Fick principle, total oxygen delivery is the product of the oxygen content of the blood and the rate of flow, usually measured as the cardiac output. Thus, oxygen transport is determined not only by the characteristics of the red cells and their number but also by pulmonary function, cardiac function, and capillary patency and density.

In the field of red cell substitutes, the oxygen transport function of the solutions is usually denoted by the position of the OEC, or P_{50}. The discussion in Chapter 4 points out that this is an extreme oversimplification. The implication of a redundant oxygen transport system, such as is found in humans, is that any one of the factors mentioned above can be altered, and compensation can occur by one or more of the other links in the chain.

How the various oxygen transport components work together can be illustrated by a model of red cell function which takes into account the ability of the heart to respond to the oxygen requirement and to the viscosity of the blood. Mixed venous PO_2 is perhaps the best indicator of the overall supply of oxygen to tissues.

The physiologic requirements for a red cell substitute will depend on the clinical setting in which it is used. Thus, attention must be paid to the oxygen requirement of the recipient (e.g., exercise, fever) and any organ damage that might be present, such as heart disease or vascular problems.

The P_{50} needs to be replaced by a more accurate indicator of the ability of a solution to deliver oxygen to tissues. This can be illustrated by the relationship between O_2 used and O_2 delivered (the oxygen extraction ratio). When the supply of oxygen drops below a certain value, compromise of organ function occurs. This "critical" PO_2 is the number we would like to know, but it is not as easy to determine as P_{50}.

Studies of oxygen transport by red cell substitutes have not been carried out to the extent desired because of the lack of suitable material for study. In the future, studies will be possible with different model derivatives of hemoglobin, or other materials which will allow investigators to study the effects of each variable on overall oxygen transport.

11.5 The Modification of Hemoglobin

Hemoglobin, free in solution, will not do as a red cell substitute. Two of the reasons for this are rapid clearance by the kidney after dimerization and high oxygen affinity, which prevents adequate tissue oxygenation. Attempts to modify hemoglobin chemically are aimed at overcoming these two problems.

The main sites for reaction on the hemoglobin molecule are at the amino-terminal amino groups and at the amino groups of lysine residues on the surface of the molecule. A few amino groups are available in the interior of the molecule. In general, modification of hemoglobin restricts the transition between the two oxy and deoxy conformations, so the oxygenation function is almost always altered in some way. For example, if hemoglobin is modified in the oxy form, high oxygen affinity is usually favored, while the reverse is usually true if the modification is carried out in the deoxy condition.

Modification of the amino terminal groups usually increases oxygen affinity and interferes with either carbon dioxide or 2,3-DPG binding since these molecules bind at the terminal groups. Although these reactions have revealed much of interest about hemoglobin structure and function the derivatives are not particularly useful as red cell substitutes because neither of the two basic problems (plasma clearance and oxygen affinity) is altered.

Derivatives of pyridoxal have been studied intensively because this molecule mimics the natural allosteric effector, 2,3-DPG. In doing so it lowers the oxygen affinity into the useful range, but the molecule can still dissociate into dimers. One derivative of pyridoxal, 2-nor-2-formyl-pyridoxal 5'-phosphate, is a bifunctional reagent that reacts in the 2,3-DPG "pocket" and links β chains. In doing so, this reagent not only reduces oxygen affinity but also interferes with dimer formation and therefore prolongs plasma retention. Unfortunately, synthesis of this reagent is tedious and expensive, and no red cell substitute product has derived from it. A similar regent, bis-pyridoxal tetraphosphate, binds at the same sites and has greater potential as a red cell substitute because the synthesis is simple.

Aldehyde groups in general can react with amino groups. Thus, a variety of polyaldehydes are used to polymerize hemoglobin. These include glutaraldehyde and the numerous reagents formed from the oxidative opening of rings of sugars and nucleatodes to form dialdehydes. Polymerized hemoglobin has a prolonged plasma retention time. The problem with the polyaldehyde reactions is that they are difficult to control. The reaction occurs by formation of a Schiff's base that must be reduced with a reagent such as sodium borohydride. The polyaldehydes that react at the surface will have free aldehyde groups, and so these molecules are free to undergo reversible aggregation and binding to other materials with reactive groups. Nevertheless, the product that has been studied most intensely at this time is hemoglobin that is first reacted with pyridoxal phosphate, then glutaraldehyde to form pyridoxylated polyhemoglobin.

Newer modification reagents have been developed recently which offer the promise of better controlled reactions. These include the diaspirin 3,5-bis(dibromosalicyl)fumarate and the monoaspirin of the same compound. The aspirin binds between α chains of hemoglobin and the monofunctional reagent to an internal lysine. Both have the effect of lowering oxygen affinity and prolonging plasma retention with a single reaction. The products of these reactions have high colloid osmotic pressure but are better characterized than the products of the polyaldehyde reactions.

An interesting and potentially useful approach to the modification of hemoglobin is the conjugation of hemoglobin to a synthetic polymer such as dextran or polyethylene glycol. These conjugates have prolonged vascular retention times and do not have the reactivity of the polyaldehyde reagents. They are therefore inherently more stable.

The supply of raw material for modified hemoglobin will become a critical problem should the products become successful. Two potential sources are animal hemoglobin and hemoglobin "manufactured" by recombinant technology. Both are receiving considerable attention, but each has its own special problems. Animal hemoglobin has the potential to become antigenic on repeated exposure, and recombinant hemoglobin must be purified from culture media. Either or both of these may ultimately be successful, but it would seem prudent to use more conventional outdated human blood as the starting material for modification until the problems of toxicity are solved.

11.6 Efficacy

Without question, hemoglobin-containing red cell substitutes *can* work; that is, they do deliver oxygen and support life in the absence of red cells. These solutions *might* work in clinical applications, but there are several problems with the data collected so far.

Efficacy studies must be performed using the hemoglobin solutions of highest possible purity. Toxicity, mainly as a result of residual red blood cell stroma, will render interpretation of results nearly impossible.

Standardization of hemoglobin solutions is essential. From the literature review presented earlier it is clear that no particular solution stands out as being more or less efficacious than the others. It appears that the only necessary qualities are near-physiologic oxygen affinity (P_{50}), a vascular retention long enough so that the deleterious effects of acute anemia do not obscure other physiologic effects, and a high enough purity so that renal toxicity is not a serious problem. A standardized solution would be one that either could be prepared by any investigator working in a reasonably equipped laboratory or one that is produced commercially and made available to any qualified investigator. Under these circumstances, data from different laboratories could be compared and evaluated properly.

Although no two investigators will ever agree completely on protocol design the literature is plagued with animal protocols that cannot be compared. It would be foolish to recommend protocol standardization, but certain basic studies could be done according to standard procedures.

11.6.1 Hemodilution

The continuous, automatic isovolemic exchange of test solutions should be carried out in the conscious rat via femoral artery and vein. Hemodynamic monitoring should include at least mean arterial pressure and heart rate. Survival and plasma retention should be followed. Other animals could be used for this simple protocol, but rats are almost universally available, and there is a substantial literature about them.

11.6.2 Resuscitation

The rapid blood removal in about fifteen minutes should be carried out in the conscious rat to a blood pressure of about 60 mm Hg via a femoral artery. Hemodynamic monitoring should include at least mean arterial pressure and heart rate. After fifteen minutes, the blood pressure should be adjusted to 60 mm Hg by adding or removing further amounts of blood. A volume of test solution, equal to that removed, should then be replaced over a period of two to three minutes. Long-term survival and plasma disappearance should be followed.

Beyond these protocols, a clinical application should be chosen and protocols should be developed to parallel these situations as clearly as possible. For example, acute resuscitation with test solution (with the volume necessary to support blood pressure) should be followed by whatever therapy is considered definitive (e.g., Ringer's lactate, blood, saline, red cells, antibiotics). This would be followed by other therapeutic interventions (e.g., respirators, oxygen, other drugs, pressors) that would be available to a patient after some period of time such as twelve hours, for instance.

Aside from validating specific hemoglobin solutions, there is little need to continue to publish in the literature the results of these "standard" protocols. Of much more importance, future work should look beyond basic efficacy, which is established, to focus on specific organ function and damage. Some studies in the isolated perfused heart and liver were discussed in this chapter, but many more studies are needed to define the short- and long-term effects on the brain and other critical organs. Toxicity and delivery of oxygen to different organs both need to be well understood before clinicians can choose to use red cell substitutes in preference to standard therapy.

The availability of solutions and their cost effectiveness are issues that cannot be settled until products are available and clinical experience is accumulated. If therapeutic benefits in clinical settings are clear-cut there is no doubt that the solutions can be made available at a reasonable cost.

11.7 Hemoglobin Metabolism

Normally, hemoglobin is removed from the circulation after the breakdown of red cells by the reticuloendothelial system. This is so efficient that only trace amounts of hemoglobin are present in the plasma. The small amount that is in the plasma is bound to haptoglobin as αβ dimers and cleared from the circulation in the kidney. Heme is degraded, mainly in the liver, to form bile pigments that eventually appear in the feces. Even in hemolytic states, these normal mechanisms are sufficient to process plasma hemoglobin, and little appears in the urine. When the plasma hemoglobin exceeds the capacity of the plasma proteins to bind it, about 128 mg/dl, hemoglobinuria occurs.

Infusions of large amounts of hemoglobin or modified hemoglobin represent a situation for which the body is not prepared; the normal processing capability is exceeded, and hemoglobin is cleared by a multitude of mechanisms. Histologic studies show that hemoglobin appears in nearly all tissues, but the organs that seem to be particular targets for accumulation are the liver and kidney, although no tissue is spared.

Free hemoglobin is filtered in the kidney because it dissociates to αβ dimers. Modification to prevent dissociation therefore has the effect of prolongation of the plasma retention; however, in this case, the clearance mechanisms are not normal. Very few studies of the clearance mechanisms and pathways of modified hemoglobin have been carried out, but those that have been done suggest that the main clearance route for heme is in bile and, ultimately, in feces.

Within the cell, whether liver, kidney, or brain, hemoglobin is taken up in vacuoles in which the globin undergoes proteolytic degradation. In this process, oxidation with hydrogen peroxide is a normal mechanism; however, in the case of hemoglobin, the interaction of iron and hydrogen peroxide can give rise to oxygen free radicals, species that may be extremely toxic. Some studies have been carried out to demonstrate that when iron binding agents such as chelators are present formation of these free radicals can be inhibited and tissue damage possibly prevented.

Whether or not heme needs to be released from hemoglobin to be toxic is still not clear, but many workers in the field believe that it need not be. In addition, there is some evidence that in acute hemorrhagic shock, free iron may increase, growth of bacteria may be stimulated, and conditions may be set for formation of oxygen radicals on reperfusion with blood or hemoglobin solution. A school of thought has grown around the concept of reperfusion injury, and advocates of this line of reasoning issue strong warnings that hemoglobin solutions may be toxic in just the clinical settings in which they might be used. Further experimental studies are needed to clarify this point.

11.8 Toxicity

In consideration of this diverse array of data collected over nearly a century on the toxicity of hemoglobin solutions, it is probable that hemoglobin is capable of manifesting a diverse array of toxic effects.

11.8.1 Renal Toxicity

Hemoglobin toxicity to the kidney is a classic model for renal failure. Studies of this model have been carried out for nearly one hundred years, and it is clear that hemoglobin is, in fact, toxic to the kidney. The mechanisms for such toxicity include obstruction of tubules with protein, renal arterial vasospasm, and direct toxicity to tubular cells. A great deal is known about the mechanisms of hemoglobin toxicity to the kidney, but it is still not clear whether this is a limiting factor in the development of red cell substitutes. A critical issue is whether or not hemoglobin needs to be filtered in the kidney to be toxic. Those advocates of polymerization of the modified protein claim that if it is not filtered toxicity is prevented. Definitive studies must await provision of solutions free of contaminants of various types, including endotoxin.

11.8.2 "Anaphylaxis/Anaphylactoid" Reactions

Acute reactions to hemoglobin are similar to the FDA classification of adverse drug reactions in which a patient is described as having the acute onset of symptoms or signs, unaccounted for by other disease processes, from at least two of the following groups: circulatory (hypotension, shock), respiratory (asthma, apnea, dyspnea, laryngeal edema, hypoventilation, laryngismus, stridor), and cutaneous (urticaria, angioedema).

In some ways, the acute reactions seen in some animals, especially rabbits and humans, are similar to the syndrome seen after protamine reversal of heparin in patients undergoing cardiopulmonary bypass. These patients experience systemic hypotension, pulmonary hypertension, and a sudden increase in upper airway pressure one to three minutes after the injection of protamine into the right atrium. Plasma levels of C_{5a} and thromboxane rise in such subjects and give rise to this anaphylactoid reaction.

Anaphylactoid reactions can result from stimulation of mononuclear cells with elaboration of substances such as thromboxane A_2 and tumor necrosis factor and can explain constriction of coronary and renal vessels, cutaneous flushing, and pulmonary hypertension. Mononuclear cell stimulation could be by hemoglobin, heme released from hemoglobin, from endotoxin either bound to hemoglobin or preexisting in the circulation, or from oxygen radicals or other tissue-derived substances released after exposure to hemoglobin. These results could be caused either by hemoglobin itself (or heme) or by contaminants present in the solutions.

11.8.3 High Plasma Protein Concentration

Effects that result from the high concentration of protein in the plasma include osmotic effects and the effects of obstruction of renal tubules after filtration of large amounts of uncross-linked hemoglobin.

11.8.4 Ischemia

Effects that can be attributed to ischemia include the results of the oxygen affinity of hemoglobin derivatives or hemoglobin itself which is too high and does not unload oxygen properly. Some histologic findings such as those in the liver could be explained in this way.

11.8.5 Protein Purity

Although the work of Rabiner and his colleagues suggested that highly purified solutions of hemoglobin had reduced toxicity, Feola showed that even trace amounts of stromal contaminants can cause problems. Now there are methods of purifying hemoglobin to a degree never before possible. It seems that the question asked by Bayliss in 1920, "Is haemolysed blood toxic?" can now be answered.

11.8.6 Vasoconstriction

Studies of the coronary, cerebral, and renal circulations have attributed many of the toxic effects of hemoglobin to vasoconstriction. Recent studies of the coronary capillary beds of the isolated perfused rabbit heart have suggested quite clearly that coronary vasoconstriction can be avoided by suitable purification of the hemoglobin derivative. However, the story is complicated by the fact that the vasoconstrictor substance is still not identified, and it may be that the effect is mediated not by a contaminant of hemoglobin solutions but by a cytokine released by the interaction of hemoglobin and phagocytes, leukocytes, or platelets.

11.8.7 Immunogenicity

Too few studies of immunogenicity are available. Of particular interest would be research that simulates multiple exposure to the solutions to see if repeated administration would pose any particular risks for patients who require multiple transfusions. The available data indicate that the more highly derivatized hemoglobin molecules are most likely to be immunogenic but that hemoglobin in general is not strongly antigenic.

Other toxic effects, such as synergism with endotoxin, inhibition of bacterial opsonization, and coagulation defects have been reported but must be studied in detail with the newer, highly purified solutions.

11.9 Evaluation of Products

No standards have been set for the evaluation of products. Still, there is a strong need for some degree of standardization even though the physical and biologic properties of the various solutions may be quite different. In Chapter 9 is suggested a list of minimal studies that should be carried out in evaluation of any product.

Some of the studies are simple, but need to be done carefully; these include recording the accurate optical absorption spectrum and measuring the oxygen capacity by a manometric method that cannot be misinterpreted or misrepresented. Some of the crucial measurements, such as oxygen affinity, still have no standardized procedures. Composition of the solutions and presence of contaminating endotoxin and phospholipid need to be established by accepted clinical measurements.

High-pressure liquid chromatography is a technique that has enjoyed wide application and improvement in recent years. Although the equipment to carry out the measurements is expensive the measurements themselves are automated and highly reproducible. The technique offers the possibility of evaluating stability during storage.

Animal studies need to be done but not necessarily all studies on all products; that is, an algorithm can be generated which will reduce the number of animal studies if certain other studies are unsatisfactory. To study efficacy, for example, a solution must pass a standard rabbit pyrogen test before infusion into larger animals. Acute toxicity in the rat should be carried out, and serial killing in the rat after a standard infusion should be done to identify the major sites of tissue deposit and/or damage. Differences in species should be studied in at least the rat, rabbit, and a third species such as pig or dog before primates are infused. Special attention should be given to vasoconstriction.

Biologic half-life must be studied in a variety of species at different dosages and rates of infusion. These variables determine the actual half-life, and the determinants of the actual time of plasma retention are not yet understood clearly. In addition to the time of disappearance, the routes of disappearance should be studied by following the fate of radio-labeled hemoglobin. The label might be in the cross-linker itself, heme, iron, or protein parts of the material.

In preparing for human studies, the protocol outlined by Savitsky (see Chapter 10) should be followed in primates. Then when human trials are undertaken, this protocol should be repeated so that results can be compared not only with those of Savitsky but also with subsequent human studies that followed the same protocol.

Efficacy studies are the most difficult to specify and must follow the intended use for the solutions. It may be impossible to design good clinical studies to evaluate usefulness in resuscitation/trauma because of the availability in this country of very prompt evacuation from scenes of trauma to major medical centers and definitive care.

11.10 Clinical Trials

At least 211 human subjects have received hemoglobin solutions either as therapy for anemia or blood loss or as clinical studies to study the metabolic fate of hemoglobin after massive intravascular hemolysis. The most significant result of these studies is the tremendous array of results, ranging from absolutely no toxic effects to complete renal failure.

Early clinical studies, before the middle 1960s, were carried out before investigators and manufacturers appreciated the fact that hemoglobin solutions needed to be rigorously purified. Thus, early trials were almost certainly carried out with solutions heavily contaminated with endotoxin or stromal material that is known to be toxic.

In the modern era, the most informative study was carried out by Savitsky and his colleagues, who used only 0.26 g/kg purified hemoglobin. In eight normal volunteers, bradycardia, hypertension, and oliguria were almost uniform findings, in spite of the fact that the same solutions caused no problems in preclinical studies.

After the Savitsky studies, Moss and his group in Chicago carried out a clinical trial with pyridoxylated polymerized hemoglobin. Their theory was that filtered hemoglobin molecules are toxic, and therefore if filtration in the kidney does not take place, that hemoglobin is nontoxic. This group developed primate models that could reproduce the Savitsky toxic findings, and they convinced themselves that their solutions were safe. Nevertheless, of six normal subjects who received the same dose as in the Savitsky study, one had a severe "allergic" reaction that remains unexplained.

As in the past, several theories exist today to explain the results of Savitsky and Moss. None is satisfactory. Work must continue to develop representative animal models that reproduce toxic effects.

The current status of research in hemoglobin-based red cell substitutes is precarious. Today it is recognized that research must be carried out using pure, well-characterized solutions. These can only be prepared using modern controlled industrial methods; the time when an isolated scientist could prepare small amounts of modified hemoglobin solutions in his general laboratory and carry out useful animal work has passed. The challenge for the future is to find ways to keep industry and academia working together so that hemoglobin-based red cell substitutes can fulfill the promise they have held for more than a century.

11.11 Conclusions

There seems to be no reasonable doubt that hemoglobin, suitably modified to prevent tetramer-dimer dissociation and to adjust oxygen affinity into the physiologic range, can transport oxygen and that in many clinical situations could substitute for red cells. Thus these solutions could eliminate the fear of viral transmission, could be capable of long-term storage, and could eliminate the alloimmunization that occurs with repeated transfusion of whole blood or red cells.

Hemoglobin-based oxygen carriers are unique in that their development over a period of almost one hundred years has still not produced a solution that is approved for human use by the FDA. This extraordinary circumstance is the reflection of the complexity of the biologic reactions to massive infusion of concentrated protein solution, bringing the oxygen carrier into contact with every cell of the body.

The molecular biology revolution tempts us to search for single, unique answers to complex questions and to ignore the older literature, especially when it is conflicting and confusing. But the massive amount of data cited in this review cannot be ignored. Much of the confusion in the older literature arises because solutions of hemoglobin were either poorly purified or poorly characterized. Thus, it is now clear that even very small amounts of contaminants (e.g., phospholipids) can have significant biologic effects. One conclusion, then, is that it is pointless to perform further biologic experiments with partially purified hemoglobin or crude hemolysates.

This review points out that certain organs may be more susceptible than others to the toxic effects of hemoglobin solutions. The renal effects, for example, have been studied for many years, and effects in the coronary circulation are well known. However, the other organs at risk are less well defined. Thus, risk for each major organ system must be assessed in a systematic way, using solutions of the highest purity.

It is not enough to produce solutions that do not demonstrate a certain type of toxicity in an animal model. Rather, the mechanisms of toxicity must be understood so that removal of an impurity or modification of hemoglobin can be done with confidence that toxicity will be reduced a priori. Despite all of the experimental literature on renal effects of hemoglobin, for example, no clear understanding of its mechanism has emerged.

The fundamental question, *Is hemoglobin toxic?* still has not been answered. On balance, the literature supports the view that purification eliminates certain toxic effects, but not enough studies have been carried out by different investigators, using high-quality solutions, to confirm this impression.

Some of the variability in the toxicity seen in human trials could be because of variations in the recipients. Little attention has been paid to such questions as underlying illness, state of the immune system, and so on. Certain effects (e.g., renal toxicity) could be more pronounced in patients with underlying renal disease, dehydration, infection, or trauma. Animal models that mimic actual clinical applications need to be developed.

In spite of the anticipated infusions of massive amounts of protein, surprisingly little is known about the metabolism of modified hemoglobin. The organ distribution of these molecules (and their components, iron and heme) must be known so that their effects on target organs at risk can be minimized. Properties such as molecular size, charge, and stability may affect their specific routes of metabolism.

Too little attention has been paid to osmotic and oncotic effects. Although much is known about maximizing oxygen delivery and plasma persistence, large gaps exist in our knowledge about fluid shifts and subsequent clinical effects.

More studies are needed to assess tissue oxygenation. Thus, in many cases it is difficult to distinguish between toxicity caused by hemoglobin or its contaminants and by hypoxia due to lowered oxygen-carrying capacity, delayed oxygen off-loading, or redistribution of blood flow.

Two issues, immunization and oxygen radical damage, remain theoretically possible but are not supported by data. More studies need to be done, with well-characterized solutions, to understand whether repeated exposure to these materials will activate the immune system and increase the risk of multiple uses. In addition, relevant animal and organ perfusion models need to be developed to demonstrate whether the formation of toxic oxygen radicals is a serious threat to the recipient of these solutions.

Clearly, there is no shortage of work to be done. It is also clear that if safe alternatives to red cells for transfusion were available, they would be used. Historically, the concept has caused little controversy. But in the push to bring products to market, the large number of problems cited above has been minimized, with the result that now unexplained toxic effects of hemoglobin solutions have slowed their further development. For these products to realize their promise there is no shortcut to understanding their biologic effects. It is not reasonable to expect that industry will solve all of the important questions. Academia, too, must play an important role, and it is likely that in tackling some of these issues new insights into protein structure-function, cell-mediated immunity, and oxygen transport mechanisms will be gained.

References

Adair, G.S. (1925a) The hemoglobin system. VI. The oxygen dissociation curve of hemoglobin. *J Biol Chem* 63:529–45.

Adair, G.S. (1925b) The osmotic pressure of hemoglobin in the absence of salts. *Proc R Soc Lond* (*A*) 109:292–300.

Adams, P.A., and M.C. Berman (1980) Kinetics and mechanism of the interaction between human serum albumin and monomeric haemin. *Biochem J* 191:95–102.

Agostoni, A., R. Stabilini, M. Perrella, P.G. Pietta, M. Pace, V. Russo, and L. Sabbioneda (1987) Functional properties of glutaraldehyde cross-linked Hb in the presence of CO_2 and/or inositol hexaphosphate (IHP) *Trans Am Soc Artif Intern Organs* 33:372–73.

Ajisaka, K., and Y. Iwashita (1980) Modification of human hemoglobin with polyethylene glycol: A new candidate for blood substitute. *Biochem Biophys Res Commun* 97:1076–81.

Alexander, B., K. Odake, D. Lawlor, and M. Swanger (1975) Coagulation, hemostasis, and plasma expanders: A quarter-century enigma. *Fed Proc* 34:1429–40.

Allen, D.W., K.F. Guthe, and J. Wyman (1950) Further studies on the oxygen equilibrium of hemoglobin. *J Biol Chem* 187:393–410.

Altruda, F., V. Poli, G. Restagno, and L. Silengo (1988) Structure of the human hemopexin gene and evidence for intron-mediated evolution. *J Mol Evol* 27:102–8.

Amberson, W.R. (1937) Blood substitutes. *Biol Rev* 12:48–86.

Amberson, W.R., J. Flexner, F.R. Steggerda, A.G. Mulder, M.J. Tendler, D.S. Pandratz, and E.P. Lang (1934–35) On the use of Ringer-Locke solutions containing hemoglobin as a substitute for normal blood in mammals. *J Cell Comp Physiol* 5:359–82.

Amberson, W.R., and R. Höber (1932) Permeability of mammalian salivary glands for organic non-electrolytes. *J Cell Comp Physiol* 2:201–21.

Amberson, W.R., J.E. Jacobs, A. Hisey, and T.V. Monke (1942) Hemoglobin-saline solutions as transfusion media. In *Blood Substitutes and Blood Transfusion* (S. Mudd and W. Thalhimer, eds) 156–69, Springfield, Ill.: Charles C Thomas.

Amberson, W.R., J.J. Jennings, and C.M. Rhode (1949) Clinical experience with hemoglobin-saline solutions. *J Appl Physiol* 1:469–89.

Amberson, W.R., A.G. Mulder, F.R. Steggerda, J. Flexner, and D.S. Pankratz (1933) Mammalian life without red blood corpuscles. *Science* 78:106–7.

Anderson, M.N., C.V. Mouritzen, and E.R. Gabrielli (1966) Mechanisms of plasma hemoglobin clearance after acute hemolysis in dogs: Serum haptoglobin levels and selective deposition in liver and kidney. *Ann Surg* 164:905–12.

Antonini, E., and M. Brunori (1971) *Hemoglobin and Myoglobin in Their Reactions with Ligands.* New York: Elsevier.

Arnone, A. (1972) X-ray diffraction study of binding of 2,3-diphosphoglycerate to human deoxyhemoglobin. *Nature* 237:146–49.

Arnone, A., R.E. Benesch, and R. Benesch (1977) Structure of human deoxyhemoglobin specifically modified with pyridoxal compounds. *J Mol Biol* 115:627–42.

Artman, M., J.D. Jackson, R.J. Boucek, T.P. Graham, and R.C. Roerth (1986) Effects of endotoxin on coronary vascular resistance in the isolated blood-perfused rabbit heart. *Circ Shock* 19:13–22.

Avissar, N., A. Inbal, E. Rabizadeh, M. Shaklia, and N. Shaklia (1984) Interaction of spectrin with hemnin disaggregates spectrin association. *Biochem Int* 8:113–20.

Ayer, G.D., and A.G. Gauld (1942) Uremia following blood transfusion. *Arch Pathol* 33:513–32.

Baker, C.C., J. DeSantis, L.D. Degutis, and A.E. Baue (1985) The impact of a trauma service on trauma care in a university hospital. *Am J Surg* 149:453–548.

Baker, S.L., and E.C. Dodds (1925) Obstruction of the renal tubules during the excretion of haemoglobin. *Br J Exp Pathol* 6:247–60.

Bakker, J.C., W.K. Bleeker, and J. VanderPlas (1986) Properties of hemoglobin interdimerically cross-linked with NFPLP. *Prog Clin Biol Res* 211:49–55.

Barcroft, J., C.A. Binger, A.V. Bock, J.H. Doggart, H.S. Forbes, G. Garrop, J.C. Meakins, and A.C. Redfield (1923) Observations upon the effect of high altitude on the physiological processes of the human body carried out in the Peruvian Andes chiefly at Cerro de Pasco. *Philos Trans R Soc Lond (Biol)* 211:351–480.

Barker, L.F. (1975) Food and Drug Administration regulations and licensure. *Fed Proc* 34:1522–24.

Barratt, J.O.W., and W. Yorke (1909) An investigation into the mechanism of production of blackwater. *Ann Trop Med Parisitol* 3:1–258.

Bass, N.M. (1988) The cellular fatty acid binding proteins: Aspects of structure, regulation, and function. *Int Rev Cytol* 111:143–184.

Baylis, C. (1987) Effects of administered thromboxanes on the intact, normal rat kidney. *Renal Physiol* 10:110–21.

Bayliss, W.M. (1920) Is haemolysed blood toxic? *Br J Exp Pathol* 1:1–8.

Beaven, G.H., S.H. Chen, A. D'Albis, and W.B. Gratzer (1974) A spectrophotometric study of the haemin-human serum albumin system. *Eur J Biochem* 41:539–46.

Becker, C.G., M. Wagner, A.P. Kaplan, and U. Muller-Eberhard (1985) Activation of factor XII-dependent pathways in human plasma by hematin and protoporphyrin. *J Clin Invest* 76:413–19.

Behringer, R.R., T.M. Ryan, M.P. Reilly, T. Asakura, R.D. Palmiter, R.L. Brinster, and T.M. Townes (1989) Synthesis of functional human hemoglobin in transgenic mice. *Science* 245:971–73.

Bellelli, A., M. Brunori, S.G. Condo, and B. Giardina (1987) Human hemoglobin cross-linked through the polyphosphate-binding site: Functional properties and evidence for conformers. *J Biol Chem* 262:2624–29.

Belzberg, H. (1989) The golden hour: The need for rapid resuscitation. *International Symposium on Red Cell Substitutes,* San Francisco, 16 May, 1989.

Benabe, J.E., S. Klahr, M.K. Hoffman, and A.R. Morrison (1980) Production of thromboxane A_2 by the kidney in glycerol-induced acute renal failure in the rabbit. *Prostaglandins* 19:333–47.

Bencowitz, H.Z., P.D. Wagner, and J.B. West (1982) Effect of change in P_{50} on exercise tolerance at high altitude: A theoretical study. *J Appl Physiol* 53:1487–95.

Benesch, R., and R.E. Benesch (1967) The effect of organic phosphates from the human erythrocyte on the allosteric properties of hemoglobin. *Biochem Biophys Res Commun* 26:162–67.

Benesch, R., and R.E. Benesch (1981) Preparation and properties of hemoglobin modified with derivatives of pyridoxal. *Methods Enzymol* 76:147–158.

Benesch, R., R.E. Benesch, and S. Kwong (1982) Labeling of hemoglobin with pyridoxal phosphate. *J Biol Chem* 257:1320–24.

Benesch, R., R.E. Benesch, S. Yung, and R. Edalji (1975) Hemoglobin covalently bridges across the polyphosphate binding site. *Biochem Biophys Res Commun* 63:1123–29.

Benesch, R., L. Triner, R.E. Benesch, S. Kwong, and M. Verosky (1984) Enhanced oxygen unloading by an interdimerically cross-linked hemoglobin in an isolated perfused rabbit heart. *Proc Natl Acad Sci USA* 81:2941–43.

Benesch, R.E., R. Benesch, R.D. Renthal, and N. Maeda (1972) Affinity labeling of the polyphosphate binding site of hemoglobin. *Biochemistry* 11:3576–82.

Benesch, R.E., and S. Kwong (1988) Bispyridoxal polyphosphates: A new class of specific intramolecular cross-linking agents for hemoglobin. *Biochem Biophys Res Commun* 156:9–14.

Benesch, R.E., and S. Kwong (1990) The stability of the heme-globin linkage in some normal, mutant, and chemically modified hemoglobins. *J Biol Chem* 265:14881–85.

Beppu, M., M. Nagoya, and K. Kikugawa (1986) Role of heme compounds in the erythrocyte membrane damage induced by lipid hydroperoxide. *Chem Pharm Bull* (Tokyo) 34:5063–70.

Bert, P. (1879) *Leçons sur la Respiration*. London: L. Baillière Tindall.

Bing, R.J. (1944) The effect of hemoglobin and related pigments on renal functions of the normal and acidotic dog. *Bull Johns Hopkins Hosp* 74:161–76.

Birndorf, N.I., and H. Lopas (1969) Evaluation of stroma-free hemoglobin solution: Effects on renal function in cynomolgus monkeys. *US Army Med Res Lab* 20:1–13.

Birndorf, N.I., H. Lopas, and S.J. Robboy (1971) Disseminated intravascular coagulation and renal failure. *Lab Invest* 25:314–19.

Biro, G.P. (1982) Comparison of acute cardiovascular effects and oxygen supply following haemodilution with dextran, stroma-free haemoglobin solution and fluorocarbon suspension. *Cardiovasc Res* 16:194–204.

Biro, G.P., and D. Beresford-Kroeger (1980) The effect of hemodilution with stroma-free hemoglobin and dextran on collateral perfusion of ischemic myocardium in the dog. *Am Heart J* 99:64–75.

Biro, G.P., D. Beresford-Kroeger, and B.V. Smith (1978) Myocardial oxygen supply during hemodilution with stroma-free hemoglobin and methemoglobin solutions. In *Blood Substitutes and Plasma Expanders* (G.A. Jamieson and T.J. Greenwalt, eds) 213–22, New York: Alan R. Liss.

Biro, G.P., G.C. Taichman, B. Lada, W.J. Keon, A.L. Rosen, and L.R. Sehgal (1988) Coronary vascular actions of stroma-free hemoglobin preparations. *Artif Organs* 12:40–50.

Bischoff, T.H.W. (1835) Beiträge zur Lehre von dem Blute und der Transfusion desselben. *Arch Anat Physiol Wissensch Med* 347.

Blackburn, C.R.B., W.J. Hensley, D.K. Grant, and F.B. Wright (1954) Studies on intravascular hemolysis in man. The pathogenesis of the initial stages of acute renal failure. *J Clin Invest* 33:825–34.

Blakowski, S.N., L.R. Zacharski, and J.R. Beck (1986) Postoperative elevation of human peripheral blood monocyte tissue factor coagulant activity. *J Lab Clin Med* 108:117–20.

Bleeker, W.K., J. VanderPlas, J. Agterberg, G. Rigter, and J.C. Bakker (1986) Prolonged vascular retention of a hemoglobin solution modified by cross-linking with 2-nor-2-formylpyridoxal 5'-phosphate. *J Lab Clin Med* 108:448–55.

Bleeker, W.K., J. VanderPlas, R.I.J. Feitsma, J. Agterberg, G. Rigter, A. deVries-van Rosen, E.K.J. Pauwels, and J.C. Bakker (1989) In vivo distribution and elimination of hemoglobin modified by intramolecular cross-linking with 2-nor-2-formylpyridoxal 5'-phosphate. *J Lab Clin Med* 113:151–61.

Blumberg, N., and T.R. Bove (1978) Uncross-matched blood for emergency transfusion: One year's experience in a civilian setting. *JAMA* 240:2057–59.

Blumenstein, J., S.C. Tam, J.E. Chang, and J.T.F. Wong (1978) Experimental transfusion of dextran-hemoglobin. In *Blood Substitutes and Plasma Expanders*. (G.A. Jamieson and T.J. Greenwalt, eds) 205–12, New York: Alan R. Liss.

Blundell, J. (1824) *Researches Physiological and Pathological*. London: E. Cox and Sons.

Bohr, C., K.A. Hasselbalch, and A. Krogh (1904) Über einen in biologischer Bezeihung wichtigen Einfluss, den die Kohlensaurespannung des Blütes auf dessen Saurstoffbindung. *Scand Arch Physiol* 16:402–12.

Bolin, R.B., D. Smith, G. Moore, G. Boswell, and F. DeVenuto (1983) Hematologic effects of hemoglobin solutions in animals. In *Advances in Blood Substitute Research* (R.A.B. Bolin, R.P. Geyer, and G.J. Nemo, eds) 117–26, New York: Alan R. Liss.

Bolton, W., and M.F. Perutz (1970) Three-dimensional Fourier synthesis of horse deoxyhemoglobin at 2 Angstrom units resolution. *Nature* 228:551–52.

Bonhard, K. (1975a) Acute oxygen supply by infusion of hemoglobin solutions. *Fed Proc* 34:1466–67.

Bonhard, K. (1975b) Experimentelle Erfahrungen mit Hämoglobin-Infusionslösungen. In *Internationales Symposium über Struktur und Function der Erythrozyten* (S. Rappaport and F. Jung, eds) 221–25, Berlin: Akademie-Verlag.

Bonhard, K. (1988) Hemoglobin preparations for perfusion and infusion problems of large-scale production. *Biomater Artif Cells Artif Organs* 16:85–91.

Bonkowsky, H.L., D.L. Tschudy, A. Collins, J. Doherty, I. Bossenmaier, R. Cardinal, and C.J. Watson (1971) Repression of the overproduction of porphyrin precursors in acute intermittent porphyria by intravenous infusions of hematin. *Proc Natl Acad Sci USA* 68:2725–29.

Bordley, J. (1931) Reactions following transfusion of blood with urinary suppression and uremia. *Arch Intern Med* 47:288–315.

Bowditch, H.P. (1871) Über die Eigenthumlichkeiten der Reizbarkeit, welche die Muskelfasern des Herzens zeigen. *Physiol Anstalt Leipzig* 6:139–76.

Brandt, J.L., R. Frank, and H.C. Lichtman (1950) Normal hemoglobin clearances in chronic proteinuria. *Proc Soc Exp Biol Med* 74:863–65.

Brandt, J.L., R. Frank, and H.C. Lichtman (1951) The effect of hemoglobin solutions on renal functions in man. *Blood* 6:1152–58.

Braun, S.R., F.R. Weiss, A.I. Keller, J.R. Ciccone, and H.G. Preuss (1970) Evaluation of the renal toxicity of heme proteins and their derivatives: A role in the genesis of acute tubule necrosis. *J Exp Med* 131:443–60.

Brinton, J.H. (1878) The transfusion of blood and the intravenous injection of milk. *Med Rec.* 14:344–47.

Brodie, T.G. (1900) The immediate action of an intravenous injection of blood serum. *J Physiol* 26:48–99.

Brown, G.L., and H.H. Dale (1936) Perfusion with a solution of hemolyzed red corpuscles. *J Physiol* 86:42–43.

Brunori, M., M. Coletta, and E. DiCera (1986) A cooperative model for ligand binding to biological macromolecules as applied to oxygen carriers. *Biophys Chem* 23:215–22.

Brunori, M., G. Falcioni, E. Fioretti, B. Giardina, and G. Rotilio (1975) Formation of superoxide in the autoxidation of the isolated α and β chains of human hemoglobin and its involvement in hemichrome precipitation. *Eur J Biochem* 53:99–104.

Bucala, R., M. Kawakami, and A. Cerami (1983) Cytotoxicity of a perfluorocarbon blood substitute to macrophages in vitro. *Science* 220:965–67.

Bucci, E., C. Fronticelli, A. Razynska, and B. Urbaitis (1989) Overview of chemically obtained oxygen carriers from hemoglobin: Pseudocross-linked tetramers. *Biomater Artif Cells Artif Organs* 17:637.

Bucci, E., A. Razynska, B. Urbaitis, and C. Fronticelli (1989) Pseudo-cross-link of human hemoglobin with mono-(3,5-dibromosalicyl)-fumarate. *J Biol Chem* 264:6191–95.

Bucher, J.R., T. Ming, and S.D. Aust (1983) The requirement for ferric in the initiation of lipid peroxidation by chelated ferrous iron. *Biochem Biophys Res Commun* 111:777–84.

Bunn, H.F. (1971) Differences in the interaction of 2,3-diphosphoglycerate with certain mammalian hemoglobins. *Science* 172:1049–50.

Bunn, H.F., W.T. Esham, and R.W. Bull (1969) The renal handling of hemoglobin. I. Glomerular filtration. *J Exp Med* 129:909–24.

Bunn, H.F., and J.H. Jandl (1967) Renal handling of hemoglobin. II. Catabolism. *J Exp Med* 129:925–34.

Bunn, H.F., and J.H. Jandl (1968a) Exchange of heme among hemoglobins and between hemoglobin and albumin. *J Biol Chem* 243:465–75.

Bunn, H.F., and J.H. Jandl (1968b) The renal handling of hemoglobin. *Trans Assoc Am Physicians* 81:147–52.

Busch, M., B. Eble, D. Heilbron, and G. Vyas (1990) Letter: Risk associated with transfusion of HIV antibody-negative blood. *N Engl J Med* 322:850–51.

Buttle, G.A.H., A. Kekwick, and A. Schweitzer (1940) Blood substitutes in treatment of acute hemorrhage. *Lancet* 2:507–10.

Bywaters, E.G.L., and D. Beall (1940) Crush injuries with impairment of renal function. *Br Med J* 1:427–32.

Cain, S.M. (1977) Oxygen delivery and uptake in dogs during hypoxic hypoxia. *J Appl Physiol* 42:228–34.

Camp, F.R. (1975) Lessons learned applicable to civil disaster: Recipient identification and blood transfusion. *J Trauma* 115:743–44.

Camp, F.R., and R.B. Dawson (1974) Prevention of injury to multiple casualties requiring resuscitation following blood loss. *Mil Med* 139:893–98.

Cannan, R.K., and J. Redish (1942) The large-scale production of crystalline human hemoglobin: With preliminary observations on the effect of its injection in man. In *Blood Substitutes and Blood Transfusion* (S. Mudd and W. Thalhimer, eds) 147–55, Springfield, Ill.: Charles C Thomas.

Carrell, R.W., C.C. Winterbourn, and E.A. Rachmilewitz (1975) Activated oxygen and haemolysis. *Br J Haematol* 30:259–64.

Carson, J.L., R.K. Spence, R.M. Poses, and G. Bonavita (1988) Severity of anaemia and operative mortality and morbidity. *Lancet* 1:727–29.

Cerny, L.C., D.M. Stasiws, and E.L. Cerny (1982) Biophysical properties of resuscitation fluids. *Crit Care Med* 10:254–60.

Chang, J.E., and J.T.F. Wong (1977) Synthesis of soluble dextran-hemoglobin complexes of different molecular sizes. *Can J Biochem* 55:398–403.

Chang, T.M.S. (1988) 30th anniversary in artificial red blood cell research. *Biomater Artif Cells Artif Organs* 16:1–9.

Chang, T.M.S. (1990) Editorial. Modified hemoglobin: Endotoxin and safety standards. *Biomater Artif Cells Artif Organs* 18:vii–viii.

Chang, T.M.S., and R. Varma (1988) Immunological and systemic effects of transfusions in rats using pyridoxylated hemoglobin and polyhemoglobin from homologous and heterogeneous sources. *Biomater Artif Cells Artif Organs* 16:205–15.

Charache, S. and C.L. Conley (1964) Rate of sickling of red cells during deoxygenation of blood from persons with various sickling disorders. *Blood* 24:25–48.

Charache, S. (1974) Hemoglobins with altered oxygen affinity. *Clinics Haematol* 3:357–81.

Chatterjee, R., E.V. Welty, R.Y. Walder, S.L. Pruitt, P.H. Rogers, A. Arnone, and J.A. Walder (1986) Isolation and characterization of a new hemoglobin derivative cross-linked between α chains (lysine 99α_1–lysine 99α_2). *J Biol Chem* 261:9929–37.

Cherfas, J. (1990) Virus-like agent blamed for mad cow disease. *Science* 247:523.

Chernoff, A.I., H.G. Klein, and L.A. Sherman (1989) Research opportunities in transfusion medicine: Report from an American Association of Blood Banks think tank. *Transfusion* 29:711–40.

Chien, S. (1977) Clinical rheology in cardiovascular disease. *Ninth European Conference on Microcirculation*, Antwerp, 1976, 472–74, Basel: Karger.

Chou, A.C., and C.D. Fitch (1981) Mechanism of hemolysis induced by ferriprotoporphyrin IX. *J Clin Invest* 68:672–77.

Christensen, S.M., F. Medina, R.M. Winslow, S.M. Snell, A. Zegna, and M.A. Marini (1988) Preparation of human hemoglobin A_0 for possible use as a blood substitute. *J Biochem Biophys Methods* 17:143–54.

Chui, D., and B. Lubin (1989) Oxidative hemoglobin denaturation and rbc destruction: The effect of heme on red cell membranes. *Semin Hematol* 26:128–35.

Clark, L.C. (1985) Introduction to fluorocarbons. *Int Anesthesiol Clin* 23:1–9

Clark, L.C., and F. Gollan (1966) Survival of mammals breathing organic liquids equilibrated with oxygen at atmospheric pressure. *Science* 152:1755–56.

Clifford, C.B., D.A. Wessels, and C.D. Smith (1989) Morphologic effects of hypervolemic administration of DBBF hemoglobin in the rat. *Biomater Artif Cells Artif Organs* 18:321–28.

Cochin, A., T.K.D. Gupta, R.D. DeWoskin, and G.S. Moss (1972) Immunogenic properties of stroma versus stroma-free hemoglobin solution. *Surg Forum* 23:19–21.

Cohen, M.V. (1989) Free radicals in ischemic and reperfusion myocardial injury: Is this the time for clinical trials? *Ann Intern Med* 111:918–31.

Cohn, E.J. (1947) The separation of blood into fractions of therapeutic value. *Ann Intern Med* 26:341–52.

Comroe, J.H. (1976) Lags between initial discovery and clinical application to cardiovascular pulmonary medicine and surgery. Appendix B, Part 1. *Report of the President's Biomedical Research Panel.* DHEW Publication (05)76–502, April 30.

Cooper, J.F. (1990) Resolving LAL test interferences. *J Parenter Sci Technol* 44:13–15.

Corcoran, A.C., and I.H. Page (1945) Renal damage from ferroheme pigments myoglobin, hemoglobin, hematin. *Tex Rep Biol Med* 3: 528–44.

Crosby, W.H., and W. Dameshek (1951) The significance of hemoglobinemia and associated hemosiderinuria, with particular reference to various types of hemolytic anemia. *J Lab Clin Med* 38:829–41.

Cumming, A.D., J.W. McDonald, R.M. Lindsay, K. Solez, and A.L. Linton (1989) The protective effect of thromboxane synthetase inhibition on renal function in systemic sepsis. *Am J Kid Dis* 13:114–19.

Cunnington, P.G., S.N. Jenkins, S.C. Tam, and J.T.F. Wong (1981) Oxygen-binding and immunological properties of complexes between dextran and animal haemoglobins. *Biochem J* 193:261–66.

Davies, M.J. (1989) Crystalloid or colloid: Does it matter? *J Clin Anes-*

thesia 1:464–71.

Dawidson, I., S. Drukker, B. Hedlund, D.H. Marks, and J. Reisch (1988) Deleterious effects of stroma-free hemoglobin used as resuscitative fluid for rats with ischemic intestinal shock. *Crit Care Med* 16:606–9.

Deen, W.M., B. Satvat, and J.M. Jamieson (1980) Theoretical model for glomerular filtration of charged solutes. *Am J Physiol* 238:F126–39.

DeGowin, E.L. (1942) Discussion of "Hemoglobin-saline solutions as transfusion media." In *Blood Substitutes and Blood Transfusion* (S. Mudd and W. Thalhimer, eds) 170, Springfield, Ill.: Charles C Thomas.

DeGowin, E.L., E.D. Warner, and W.L. Randall (1938) Renal insufficiency from blood transfusion. II. Anatomic changes in man compared with those in dogs with experimental hemoglobinuria. *Arch Intern Med* 61:609–30.

Demaria, W.J.A., and J.S. Harris (1955) Effect of magnesium sulfate on the alterations in renal dynamics induced by intravenous hemoglobin. *Am J Physiol* 182:251–55.

DeNavasquez, S. (1940) The excretion of hemoglobin, with special reference to the "transfusion" kidney. *J Pathol Bacteriol* 5:413–25.

DeVenuto, F. (1982a) Hemoglobin solutions as oxygen-delivering resuscitation fluids. *Crit Care Med* 10:238–45.

DeVenuto, F. (1982b) Oxygen-carrying resuscitation solutions. *Crit Care Med* 10:237 (abstr).

DeVenuto, F. (1988) Evaluation of human and bovine modified hemoglobin solution as oxygen-carrying fluid blood volume replacement. *Biomater Artif Cells Artif Organs* 16:77–83.

DeVenuto, F., K.R. Busse, and A.I. Zegna (1981) Oxygen transport after hemodilution of human blood with crystalline hemoglobin solution. *Surg Gynecol Obstet* 153:332–36.

DeVenuto, F., H.I. Friedman, and P.W. Mellick (1980) Massive exchange transfusions with crystalline hemoglobin solution and blood volume. *Surgery* 151:361–65.

DeVenuto, F., H.I. Friedman, R.J. Neville, and C.C. Peck (1979) Appraisal of hemoglobin solution as a blood substitute. *Surg Gynecol Obstet* 149:417–36.

DeVenuto, F., W.Y. Moores, A.I. Zegna, and T.F. Zuck (1977) Total and partial blood exchange in the rat with hemoglobin prepared by crystallization. *Transfusion* 17:555–62.

DeVenuto, F., and A. Zegna (1982) Blood exchange with pyridoxylated and polymerized hemoglobin solution. *Surg Gynecol Obstet* 155:342–46.

DeVenuto, F., and A. Zegna (1983) Preparation and evaluation of pyridoxylated-polymerised human haemoglobin. *J Surg Res* 34:205–12.

DeVenuto, F., and A.I. Zegna (1981) Transfusion with pyridoxylated-polymerized hemoglobin solutions. *Transfusion* 21:599.

DeVenuto, F., A.I. Zegna, and K.R. Busse (1979) Lyophilization of crystalline hemoglobin solution and exchange transfusions with lyophilized, reconstituted hemoglobin. *Surg Gynecol Obstet* 148:69–75.

DeVenuto, F., T.F. Zuck, A.I. Zegna, and W.Y. Moores (1977) Characteristics of stroma-free hemoglobin prepared by crystallization. *J Lab Clin Med* 89:509–16.

Diamond, L. (1980) A history of blood transfusion. In *Blood, Pure and Simple* (M.M. Wintrobe, ed) 659–90, New York: McGraw-Hill.

Diamond, L.K. (1965) History of blood banking in the United States. *JAMA* 193:128–32.

DiCera, E., C.H. Robert, and S.J. Gill (1987) Allosteric interpretation of the oxygen-binding reaction of human hemoglobin tetramers. *Biochemistry* 26:4003–8.

Djordjevich, L., J. Mayoral, and A. Ivankovich (1985) Synthetic erythrocytes: Cardiorespiratory changes during exchange transfusions. *Anesthesiology* 63:109 (abstr).

Dormandy, T.L. (1978) Harvey at 400. *Lancet* 1:708.

Drummond, G.S. (1989) Control of heme catabolism by Sn-protoporphyrin. *Semin Hematol* 26:24–26.

Dunphy, J.E., and J.G.I. Gibson (1943) Effect of infusions of bovine serum albumin in experimental shock. *Surgery* 14:509–18.

Eaton, J.W., P. Brandt, and J.R. Mahoney (1982) Hemoglobin: A natural bacteriostat. *Science* 215:691–93.

Eaton, J.W., T.D. Skelton, and E. Berger (1974) Survival at extreme altitude: Protective effect of increased hemoglobin-oxygen affinity. *Science* 185:743–44.

Elert, O., and U. Otterman (1979) Cardioplegic hemoglobin perfusion: A method of providing optimal myocardial protection. *Thorac Cardiovasc Surg* 27:245–47.

Elia, D., H.J. Sternberg, A. Greenburg, and G.W. Peskin (1974) Stroma-free hemoglobin in the resuscitation of hemorrhagic shock. *Surg Forum* 25:201–04.

Engerson, T.D., T.G. McKelvey, D.B. Rhyne, E.B. Boggio, S.J. Snyder, and H.P. Jones (1987) Conversion of xanthine dehydrogenase to oxidase in ischemic rat tissues. *J Clin Invest* 79:1564–70.

Estep, T.N., M.K. Bechtel, S.L. Bush, T.J. Miller, S. Szeto, and L.E. Webb (1989) The purification of hemoglobin solutions by heating. In *The Red Cell: Seventh Ann Arbor Conference* (G. Brewer, ed) 325–38, New York: Alan R. Liss.

Estep, T.N., M.K. Bechtel, T.J. Miller, and A. Bagdasarian (1988) Virus inactivation in hemoglobin solutions by heat. *Biomater Artif Cells Artif Organs* 16:129–34.

Faasen, A.E., R. Sundby, S.S. Panter, R.M. Condie, and B.E. Hedlund (1988) Hemoglobin: A livesaver and an oxidant. How to tip the balance. *Biomater Artif Cells Artif Organs* 16:93–104.

Fairly, N.H. (1940) The fate of extracorpuscular circulating hemoglobin. *Br J Med* 2:213–17.

Fantl, W., L.R. Manning, H. Ueno, A. DiDonato, and M. Manning (1987) Properties of carboxymethylated cross-linked hemoglobin A. *Biochemistry* 26:5755–61.

Fantl, W.J., A.D. Donato, J.M. Manning, P.H. Rogers, and A. Arnone (1987) Specifically carboxymethylated hemoglobin as an analogue of carbamino hemoglobin: Solution and x-ray studies of carboxymethylated hemoglobin and x-ray studies of carbamino hemoglobin. *J Biol Chem* 26:12700–13.

Feola, M., D. Azar, and L. Wiener (1979) Improved oxygenation of ischemic myocardium by hemodilution with stroma-free hemoglobin solution. *Chest* 75:369–75.

Feola, M., H. Gonzalez, P.C. Canizaro, D. Bingham, and P. Periman (1983) Development of a bovine stroma-free hemoglobin solution as a blood substitute. *Surg Gynecol Obstet* 157:399–408.

Feola, M., J. Simoni, P.C. Canizaro, R. Tran, G. Raschbaum, and F.J. Behal (1988) Toxicity of polymerized hemoglobin solutions. *Surg Gynecol Obstet* 166:–22.

Feola, M., J. Simoni, R. Tran, and P.C. Canizaro (1988) Mechanisms of toxicity of hemoglobin solutions. *Biomater Artif Cells Artif Organs* 16:217–26.

Fish, R.E., A.H. Burns, C.H. Lang, and J.A. Spitzer (1985) Myocardial dysfunction in a nonlethal, nonshock model of chronic endotoxemia. *Circ Shock* 16:241–52.

Fitch, C.D., R. Chevli, P. Kanjananggulpan, P. Dutta, K. Chevli, and A.C. Chou (1983) Intracellular ferriprotoporphyrin IX is a lytic agent. *Blood* 62:1165–68.

Flink, E.B. (1947) Blood transfusion studies. III. The relationship of hemoglobinemia and of the pH of the urine to renal damage produced by injection of hemoglobin solutions into dogs. *J Lab Clin Med* 32:223–61.

Friedman, H.I., and F. DeVenuto (1982) Morphological effects of transfusions with hemoglobin solutions. *Crit Care Med* 10:288–93.

Friedman, H.I., F. DeVenuto, L. Lollini, P. Mellick, and T.F. Zuck (1978) Morphologic effects following massive exchange transfusions with a stroma-free hemoglobin solution. I. Liver. *Lab Invest* 39:167–77.

Friedman, H.I., F. DeVenuto, L. Lollini, P. Mellick, and T.F. Zuck (1979) Morphologic effects following massive exchange transfusions with a stroma-free hemoglobin solution. II. Kidney. *Lab Invest* 40:655–67.

Friedman, H.I., F. DeVenuto, B.D. Schwartz, and T.J. Nemeth (1984) In vivo evaluation of pyridoxylated-polymerized hemoglobin solution. *Surgery* 159:429–35.

Friedman, H.I., F. DeVenuto, T.F. Zuck, P. Mellick, and L. Lollini (1977) Histologic and ultrastructural effects of stroma-free hemoglobin solutions on rat liver, kidney and brain. *Surg Forum* 28:3–5.

Fronticelli, C., E. Bucci, and C. Orth (1984) Solvent regulation of oxygen affinity in hemoglobin. *J Biol Chem* 259:10841–44.

Fronticelli, C., T. Sato, C. Orth, and E. Bucci (1986) Bovine hemoglobin as a potential source of hemoglobin-based oxygen carriers: Cross-linking with bis(2,3-dibromosalicyl)fumarate. *Biochim Biophys Acta* 874:76–81.

Fukumoto, S., and K. Tanaka (1983) Protective effects of thromboxane A_2 synthetase inhibitors on endotoxin shock. *Prostaglandins Leukotrienes Med* 11:179–88.

Garby, L., and W.D. Noyes (1959) Studies on hemoglobin metabolism. I. The kinetic properties of the plasma hemoglobin pool in normal man. *J Clin Invest* 38:1479–83.

Gendler, E., S. Gendler, and M.E. Nimni (1984) Toxic reactions evoked by glutaraldehyde-fixed pericardium and cardiac valve tissue bioprosthesis. *J Biomed Mater Res* 18:727–36.

George, P. and A. Schejter (1964) The reactivity of ferrocytochrome C with iron-binding ligands. *J Biol Chem* 239:1504–8.

Geyer, R.P. (1975) Potential uses of artificial blood substitutes. *Fed Proc* 34:1525–28.

Geyer, R.P., R.G. Monroe, and K. Taylor (1968) Survival of rats having red cells totally replaced with emulsified fluorocarbon. *Fed Proc* 27:384.

Gill, S.J., E. DiCera, M.L. Doyle, G.A. Bishop, and C.H. Robert (1987) Oxygen binding constants for human hemoglobin tetramers. *Biochemistry* 26:3995–4002.

Gilligan, D.R., M.D. Altschule, and E.M. Katersky (1941) Studies of hemoglobinemia and hemoglobinuria produced in man by intravenous injection of hemoglobin solutions. *J Clin Invest* 20:177–87.

Gilroy, D., C. Shaw, E. Parry, and W. Odling-Smee (1989) Detection of a vasoconstrictor factor in stroma-free haemoglobin solutions. *J Trauma* 28:1312–16.

Goldberg, M. (1962) Studies of acute renal effects of hemolyzed red blood cells in dogs including estimations of renal blood flow with krypton. *J Clin Invest* 41:2112–22.

Goldberg, M.A., S.P. Dunning, and H.F. Bunn (1988) Regulation of the erythropoietin gene: Evidence that the oxygen sensor is a heme protein. *Science* 242:1412–15.

Goldfinger, D. (1977) Uncross-matched blood for emergency transfusion. *JAMA* 237:1826–27.

Goodnough, T.L., S. Rudnick, T.H. Price, S.K. Ballas, M.L. Collins, J.P. Crowley, M. Kosmin, M.S. Kruskall, B.A. Lenes, J.E. Menitove, L.E. Silberstein, K.J. Smith, C.H. Wallas, R. Abels, and M.V. Tress (1989) Increased preoperative collection of autologous blood with recombinant human erythropoietin therapy. *N Engl J Med* 321:1163–68.

Goodwin, W.E., E.F. Alston, and J.H. Semens (1950) Hematuria and sickle cell disease: Unexplained, gross unilateral, renal hematuria in Negroes, coincident with the blood in sickling trait. *J Urol* 63:79–96.

Goslinga, H. (1981) *The Role of Blood Viscosity in Hemodilution and Shock.* Heidelberg: Springer-Verlag.

Gould, S., L.R. Sehgal, A.L. Rosen, S.A. Gould, R. DeWoskin, and G.S. Moss (1988) Characteristics of polymerized pyridoxylated hemoglobin. *Biomater Artif Cells Artif Organs* 16:173–83.

Gould, S.A., A.L. Rosen, L. Sehgal, G. Noud, H. Sehgal, R. DeWoskin, H. Levine, M. Kerstein, C. Rice, and G.S. Moss (1980) The effect of altered haemoglobin-oxygen affinity on oxygen transport by haemoglobin solution. *J Surg Res* 28:246–51.

Gould, S.A., A.L. Rosen, L.R. Sehgal, H.L. Sehgal, L.A. Langdale, L.M. Krause, C.L. Rice, and W.H. Chamberlin (1986) Fluosol-DA as a red-cell substitute in acute anemia. *N Engl J Med* 314:1653–56.

Gould, S.A., A.L. Rosen, L.R. Sehgal, H.L. Sehgal, and G.S. Moss (1986) Polymerized pyridoxylated hemoglobin: Efficacy as an oxygen carrier. *J Trauma* 26:903–8.

Gould, S.A., L.R. Sehgal, A.L. Rosen, H.L. Sehgal, and G.S. Moss (1986) The development of polymerized pyridoxylated hemoglobin solution as a red cell substitute. *Ann Emerg Med* 15:1416–19.

Greenburg, A.G., K. Ginsburg, and G.W. Peskin (1977) Preservation of stroma-free hemoglobin solution. *Surg Forum* 28:5–7.

Greenburg, A.G. and P.W. Maffuid (1983) Modification of hemoglobin-ring opened dials. In *Progress in Clinical and Biological Research: Advances in Blood Substitute Research* (R.B. Bolin, R.P. Geyer, and G.J. Nemo, eds) 9–17, New York: Alan R. Liss.

Greenburg, A.G., G.W. Peskin, D.B. Hoyt, and W.Y. Moores (1982) Is it necessary to improve the intravascular retention of hemoglobin solutions? *Crit Care Med* 10:266–69.

Greenburg, A.G., M. Schooley, K.A. Ginsburg, and G.W. Peskin (1978) Pyridoxylated stroma-free hemoglobin in resuscitation of hemorrhagic shock. *Surg Forum* 29:44–46.

Grisham, M.B. (1985) Myoglobin-catalyzed hydrogen peroxide dependent arachidonic acid peroxidation. *J Free Rad Biol Med* 1:227–32.

Guillochon, D., M.W. Vijayalakshmi, A. Sow-Thiam, and D. Thomas (1986) Effect of glutaraldehyde on hemoglobin: functional aspects and Mössbauer parameters. *Biochemistry* 64:29–37.

Gunnar, W., O. Jonasson, G. Merlotti, J. Stone, and J. Barrett (1987)

Head injury and hemorrhagic shock: Studies of the blood brain barrier and intracranial pressure after resuscitation with normal saline solution, 3% saline solution and dextran 40. *Surgery* 103:398–407.

Guthrie, C.C., and F.G. Pike (1907) The relation of the activity of the excised mammalian heart to pressure in the coronary vessels and to its nutrition. *Am J Physiol* 18:14–38.

Gutierrez, G. (1988) The relationship of tissue oxygenation to cellular bioenergetics. *Adv Exp Med Biol* 227:183–205.

Gutteridge, J.M.C., R. Richmond, and B. Halliwell (1979) Inhibition of the iron-catalysed formation of hydroxyl radicals from superoxide and of lipid peroxidation by desferrioxamine. *Biochem J* 184:469–72.

Guyton, A.C., C.E. Jones, and T.G. Coleman (1973) *Cardiac Output and Its Regulation*, 2nd ed. Philadelphia: Saunders.

Hales, C.A., L. Sonne, M. Peterson, D. Kong, M. Miller, and W.D. Watkins (1981) Role of thromboxane and prostacyclin in pulmonary vasomotor changes after endotoxin in dogs. *J Clin Invest* 68:497–505.

Halliwell, B., and J.M.C. Gutteridge (1984) Oxygen toxicity, oxygen radicals, transition metals and disease. *Biochem J* 219:1–14.

Halliwell, B., and J.M.C. Gutteridge (1989) *Free Radicals in Biology and Medicine*, 2nd ed, 160. Oxford: Clarendon Press.

Halsted, W.S.S. (1891) The management of wounds with especial reference to the value of blood clot in the management of dead spaces. *Johns Hopkins Hosp Rep* 2:255–62.

Hamilton, P.B., L.E. Farr, A. Hiller, and D.D. VanSlyke (1947) Preparation of hemoglobin solutions for intravenous infusion. *J Exp Med* 86:455–63.

Hamilton, P.B., A. Hiller, and D.D. VanSlyke (1947) Renal effects of hemoglobin infusions in dogs in hemorrhagic shock. *J Exp Med* 86:477–87.

Harrison, H.E., H. Bunting, N.K. Ordway, and W.S. Albrink (1947) The pathogenesis of the renal injury produced in the dog by hemoglobin or methemoglobin. *J Exp Med* 86:339–56.

Hartmann, A.F., and M.J.E. Senn (1932) Studies in edema, with particular reference to the therapeutic value of acacia. *Trans Am Pediatric Soc* 44:56–61.

Harvey, W. (1653) *Exercitatio Anatomica de Motu Cordis et Sanguinis in Animalibus*, 86, London: Leach.

Haupt, A.S., R. Ochs, and G.E. Schubert (1982) Renal lesions in ischaemic kidneys infused with haemoglobin: An electron microscopic study. *Urol Res* 10:1–6.

Hauser, C.J., C. Kaufman, R. Frantz, C. Shippy, S. Schwartz, and W.C. Shoemaker (1982) Use of crystalline hemoglobin as replacement of rbc mass. *Arch Surg* 117:782–86.

Hauser, C.J., and W.C. Shoemaker (1982) Hemoglobin solution in the treatment of hemorrhagic shock. *Crit Care Med* 10:283–87.

Hawkins, W.B. and A.C. Johnson (1939) Bile pigment and hemoglobin interrelation in anemic dogs. *Am J Physiol* 126:326–36.

Hebbel, R.P., J.W. Eaton, M. Balasingham, and M.H. Steinberg (1982) Spontaneous oxygen radical generation by sickle erythrocytes. *J Clin Invest* 70:1253–59.

Hebbel, R.P., J.W. Eaton, R.S. Kronenberg, E.D. Zanjani (1978) Human llamas. Adaptation to altitude in subjects with high hemoglobin oxygen affinity. *J Clin Invest* 162:593–600.

Hedlund, B.E. (1988) Inclusion of antioxidants in resuscitation fluids. *Basic Life Sci* 49:627–29.

Henderson, Y., and H.W. Haggard (1922) Hemorrhage as a form of asphyxia. *JAMA* 78:697–704.

Hess, J.R., S.O. Fadare, L.S.L. Tolentino, N.R. Bangal, and R.M. Winslow (1989) The intravascular persistence of cross-linked human hemoglobin. In *The Red Cell: Seventh Ann Arbor Conference* (G. Brewer, ed) 351–360, New York: Alan R. Liss.

Hill, A.V. (1910) The possible effects of the aggregation of the molecules of hemoglobin on its oxygen dissociation curve. *J Physiol Lond* 40:4–7.

Hirst, D.G., P.J. Wood, and H.C. Schwartz (1987) The modification of hemoglobin affinity for oxygen and tumor radiosensitivity by antilipidemic drugs. *Radiat Res* 112:164–72.

Hoffman, S.J., D.L. Looker, J.M. Roerich, P.E. Cozart, S.L. Durfee, J.L. Tedesco, and G.L. Steeler (1990) Expression of fully functional human hemoglobin in *Escherichia coli*. *Proc Natl Acad Sci USA*, 87:8521–25.

Holdefer, W.F., and E.A. Dowling (1974) Experimental use of heterologous stroma-free hemoglobin solution (SFHS) as a whole blood substitute. *J Surg Oncol* 6:451–59.

Hollingsworth, M.W. (1928) Blood transfusion by Richard Lower in 1665. *Ann Med Hist* 10:213–25.

Hoyt, D.B., A.G. Greenburg, G.W. Peskin, S. Forbes, and H. Reese (1980) Hemorrhagic shock and resuscitation: Improved survival with pyridoxylated stroma-free hemoglobin. *Surg Forum* 31:15–17.

Hrkal, Z., Z. Vodrazka, and I. Kalousek (1974) Transfer of heme from ferrihemoglobin and ferrihemoglobin-isolated chains to hemopexin. *Eur J Biochem* 43:73–78.

Hsia, C., S.S. Er, K. Hronowski, K. Perasud, and M.R. Ansari (1986) ATP-hemoglobin purification by ATP-affinity chromatography. *J Chromatogr* 381:153–57.

Hsia, C.J.C. (1989) Fine tuning of polymerized pyridoxylated hemoglobin as a red blood cell substitute. In *The Red Cell: Seventh Ann Arbor Conference* (G. Brewer, ed) 339–49, New York: Alan R. Liss.

Hsia, J.C., and E.R. Song S (1988) Quality control of hemoglobin-based blood substitutes. *Biomater Artif Cells Artif Organs* 16: 105–11.

Humphrey, P.R.D., J.L. Marshall, R.W. RossRussell, G. Wetherley-Mein, G.H. DuBoulay, T.C. Pearson, L. Symon, and E. Zulkha (1979) Cerebral blood-flow and viscosity in relative polycythaemia. *Lancet* 2:873–77.

Humphries, R.G., P.G. Killingback, J. Mann, J. Sempik, and J. Wilson (1981) Exchange transfusion with dextran-hemoglobin, hemoglobin, and dextran solutions in anesthetized cats. *Br J Pharmacol* 74:266P.

Hunt, C.A., R.R. Burnette, R.D. MacGregor, A.E. Strubbe, D.T. Lau, N. Taylor, and H. Kawada (1985) Synthesis and evaluation of a prototypal artificial red cell. *Science* 230:1165–68.

Hustin, A. (1914) Principe d'une nouvelle methode de transfusion muqueuse. *J Med Brux* 12:436–39.

Iwai, T., S. Sato, Y. Yamada, Y. Muraoka, K. Sakurazawa, Y. Inoue, H. Kinoshita, and M. Endo (1989) A new treatment for ischemic ulcers: Foot bath therapy using high oxygen soluble fluid. *J Cardiovasc Surg* 30:490–93.

Iwasaki, K., K. Ajisaka, and Y. Iwashita (1983) Modification of human hemoglobin with polyethylene glycol: A new candidate for blood substitute. *Biochem Biophys Res Commun* 113:513–18.

Iwasaki, K., T. Takahashi, P.S. Malchesky, H. Hiroaki, Y. Iwashita, and Y. Nose (1989) Pyridoxylated-hemoglobin-polyoxyethylene conjugate (PHP) as an oxygen carrier. *Biomater Artif Cells Artif Organs* 17:635.

Jaenike, J.R. (1966) The renal lesion associated with hemoglobinemia. I. Its production and functional evaluation in the rat. *J Exp Med* 123:523–35.

Jaenike, J.R. (1967) The renal lesion associated with hemoglobinemia: A study of the pathogenesis of the excretory defect in the rat. *J Clin Invest* 46:378–87.

Jaenike, J.R., and E.E. Schneeberger (1966) The renal lesion associated with hemoglobinemia. II. Its structural characteristics in the rat. *J Exp Med* 123:537–45.

Jennings, C.E. (1885) The intravenous injection of milk. *Br Med J* 1:1147–49.

Jesch, F.H., W. Peters, J. Hobbhahn, M. Schoenberg, and K. Messmer (1982) Oxygen-transporting fluids and oxygen delivery with hemodilution. *Crit Care Med* 10:270–74.

Jones, H.W., and G. Mackmul (1928) The influence of James Blundell on the development of blood transfusion. *Ann Med Hist* 10:242–48.

Jones, R.T., C. Head, T. Fujita, A. Grant, and R. Kluger (1989) Structural studies of hemoglobin modified with dicarboxylic acid bis(methylphosphate) cross-linking reagents. *Biomater Artif Cells Artif Organs* 17:643 (abstr).

Kaartinen, V. and I. Monnen (1988) Hemoglobin binding to deglycosylated haptoglobin. *Biochim Biophys Acta* 953:345–52.

Kanner, J., and S. Harel (1985) Initiation of membranal lipid peroxidation by activated metmyoglobin and methemoglobin. *Arch Biochem Biophys* 237:314–321.

Keipert, P.E., A.J. Aderiran, S. Kwong, and R.E. Benesch (1989) Functional properties of a new cross-linked hemoglobin designed for use as a red cell substitute. *Transfusion* 29:768–73.

Keipert, P.E., and T.M.S. Chang (1985) Pyridoxylated polyhemoglobin as a red cell substitute for resuscitation of lethal hemorrhagic shock in conscious rats. *Biomater Med Devices Artif Organs* 13:1–15.

Keipert, P.E., and T.M.S. Chang (1987) Effects of partial and total isovolemic exchange transfusion in fully conscious rats using pyridoxylated polyhemoglobin solution as a colloidal oxygen-delivering blood replacement fluid. *Vox Sang* 53:7–14.

Keipert, P.E., and L. Triner (1989) Catabolism and excretion of cross-linked hemoglobin. In *The Red Cell: Seventh Ann Arbor Conference* (G. Brewer, ed) 383–405, New York: Alan R. Liss.

Keipert, P.E., M. Verosky, and L. Triner (1988) Metabolism, distribution, and excretion of HbXL: A nondissociating interdimerically cross-linked hemoglobin with exceptional oxygen off-loading capability. *Biomater Artif Cells Artif Organs* 16:643–645.

Keipert, P.E., M. Verosky, and L. Triner (1989) Plasma retention and metabolic fate of hemoglobin modified with an interdimeric covalent cross-link. *Trans Am Soc Artif Intern Organs* 35:153–59.

Kilmartin, J.V., J. Fogg, and L. Rossi-Bernardi (1975) Identification of the high and low affinity CO_2-binding sites of human haemoglobin. *Nature* 256:759–61.

Kilmartin, J.V., and L. Rossi-Bernardi (1973) Interaction of hemoglobin with hydrogen ions, carbon dioxide, and organic phosphates. *Physiol Rev* 53:836–90.

Klein, H.G. (1989) Current trends in the use of red cells. *Biomater Artif Cells Artif Organs* 17:625.

Klotz, I.M (1971) Hemerythrin. *Subunits Biol Syst* 5:55–103.

Kohler,W. and O. Prokop (1978) Relationship between haptoglobin and *Streptococcus pyògenes* T4 antigens. *Nature* 271:373.

Kramer, G.C., P.R. Perron, D.C. Lindsey, H.S. Ho, R.A. Gunther, W.A. Boyle, and J.W. Holcroft (1986) Small-volume resuscitation with hypertonic saline dextran solution. *Surgery* 100:239–47.

Kreimeier, U., and K. Messmer (1987) New perspectives in resuscitation and prevention of multiple organ system failure. In *Surgical Research: Recent Concepts and Results* (A. Baethmann and K. Messmer, eds) 39–50, Heidelberg: Springer-Verlag.

Kremen, A.J., H. Hall, H.K. Koschnitzke, B. Stevens, and O.H. Wangensteen (1942) Studies on the intravenous administration of whole bovine plasma and serum to man. *Surgery* 11:333–55.

Kronecker, H., and W. Stirling (1875) *Beitrage zur Anatomie und Physiologie als Festgabe Carl Ludwig gewidmet.* Leipzig.

Labrude, P., C. Vigneron, E. Dellacherie, and J.L. Tayot (1988) Preparation and comparison of transfusional capacity of six stroma-free hemoglobin solutions by a hemorrhagic shock in Wistar rats. *Biomater Artif Cells Artif Organs* 16:671–72.

Lalich, J.J. (1952) The influence of in vitro hemoglobin modification on hemoglobinuric nephrosis in rabbits. *J Lab Clin Med* 40:102–10.

Lalich, J.J. (1955) The role of oxyhemoglobin and its derivatives in the pathogenesis of experimental hemoglobinuric nephrosis. *Am J Pathol* 31:153–75.

Lalla, F.R., J. Ning, and T.M.S. Chang (1989) Effects of pyridoxylated polyhemoglobin and stroma-free hemoglobin on ADP-induced platelet aggregation. *Biomater Artif Cells Artif Organs* 17:363–69.

Lamson, P.D., B.H. Robbins, and M.E. Greig (1945) Studies on shock induced by hemorrhage. *J Pharmacol Exp Ther* 8:225–34.

Landois, L. (1875) *Die Transfusion des Blutes.* Leipzig: Vogel.

Landsteiner, E.K., and C.A. Finch (1947) Hemoglobinemia accompanying transurethral resection of the prostate. *N Engl J Med* 237:310–12.

Landsteiner, K. (1901) Über agglutinationserscheinungen normalen menschlichen Blutes. *Wien Klin Wochenschr* 14:1132–34.

Lathem, W. (1959) The renal excretion of hemoglobin: Regulatory mechanisms and differential excretion of free and protein-bound hemoglobin. *J Clin Invest* 38:652–58.

Lathem, W., B.B. Davis, P.H. Zweig, and R. Dew (1960) The demonstration and localization of renal tubular reabsorption of hemoglobin by stop flow analysis. *J Clin Invest* 39:840–45.

Lathem, W., and W.E. Worley (1959) The distribution of extracorpuscular hemoglobin in circulating plasma. *J Clin Invest* 38:474–83.

Laver, M.E., P. Boysen, and K.E. Morris (1975) Water-soluble cross-linked polymerised haemoglobin free of stroma used as a blood substitute. U.S. Patent 554–051.

Lee, R., N. Atsumi, E.E. Jacobs, W.G. Austen, and G.J. Vlahakes (1989) Ultrapure, stroma-free, polymerized bovine hemoglobin solution: Evaluation of renal toxicity. *J Surg Res* 47:407–11.

Lenfant, C., and K. Sullivan (1971) Adaptation to high altitude. *N Engl J Med* 284:1298–1309.

Leonard, M., and E. Dellacherie (1984) Acylation of human hemoglobin with polyoxyethylene derivatives. *Biochim Biophys Acta* 791:219–25.

Levi, A.J., Z. Gatmaitan, and I.M. Arias (1969) Two hepatic cytoplasmic protein fractions, Y and Z, and their possible role in the hepatic uptake of bilirubin, sulfobromophthaleine, and other anions. *J Clin Invest* 48:2156–67.

Lieberthal, W., W.M. Vogel, C.S. Apstein, and C.R. Valeri (1989) Studies of the mechanism of the vasoconstrictor activity of stroma-free hemoglobin in the isolated perfused rat kidney and rabbit heart. In *The Red Cell: Seventh Ann Arbor Conference* (G. Brewer, ed) 407–422, New York: Alan R. Liss.

Lindeboom, G.A. (1954) The story of a blood transfusion to a Pope. *J Hist Med Allied Sci* 9:455–9.

Loutit, J.F., and P.L. Mollison (1943) Advantages of a disodium-citrate-glucose mixture as a blood preservative. *Br Med J* 2:744–45.

Macdonald, V.W. (1989) Methemoglobin-induced decrease of vascular reactivity to human stroma-free hemoglobin in isolated perfused rabbit hearts. In *The Red Cell: Seventh Ann Arbor Conference* (G. Brewer, ed) 423–34, New York: Alan R. Liss.

Macdonald, V.W. (1990) Comparison of oxygen delivery by hemoglobin solutions with different oxygen affinity. *J Appl Physiol* in press, 1991.

Macdonald, V.W., R.M. Winslow, M.A. Marini, and M.T. Klinker (1989) Coronary vasoconstrictor activity of purified and modified human hemoglobin. *Biomater Artif Cells Artif Organs* 18:263–82.

Maluf, N.S.R. (1949) Factors inducing renal shut-down from lysed erythrocytes: An experimental study. *Ann Surg* 130:49–67.

Mandel, M.A. (1986) Autotransfusion in elective plastic surgical operations. *Plast Reconstr Surg* 77:767–71.

Maningas, P.A., L.R. DeGuzman, F.J. Tillman, C.S. Hinson, K.J. Priegnitz, K.A. Volk, and R.F. Bellamy (1986) Small-volume infusion of 7.5% NaCl in 6% dextran 70 for the treatment of severe hemorrhagic shock in swine. *Ann Emerg Med* 15:1131–1137.

Manning, J.M. (1981) Preparation of hemoglobin carbamylated at specific NH_2-terminal residues. *Methods Enzymol* 76:159–67.

Manning, J.M., W.J. Fantl, L.R. Manning, and H.Ueno (1989) Carboxymethylated cross-linked hemoglobin A. *Biomater Artif Cells Artif Organs* 17:639.

Mansouri, A., and K.H.Winterhalter (1973) Nonequivalence of chains in hemoglobin oxidation. *Biochemistry* 12:4946–49.

Marini, M.A., G.L. Moore, R.M. Fishman, R. Jessee, F. Medina, S. Snell, and A.I. Zegna (1989) A critical examination of the reaction of pyridoxal 5'-phosphate with human hemoglobin A_0. *Biopolymers* 28:2071–83.

Marini, M.A., G.L. Moore, R.M. Fishman, R. Jesse, F. Medina, S.M. Snell, and A.I. Zegna (1990) Reexamination of the polymerization of pyridoxylated hemoglobin with glutaraldehyde. *Biopolymers* 29:71–882.

Marks, D.H., J.E. Lynett, R.M. Letscher, R.P. TenEyck, A.D. Schaerle, G.T. Makovec, and F. Medina (1987) Pyridoxylated polymerized stroma-free hemoglobin solution (SFHS-PP) as an oxygen-carrying fluid replacement for hemorrhagic shock in dogs. *Milit Med* 152: 265–71.

Marks, D.H., G.L. Moore, F. Medina, G. Boswell, L.R. Zieske, R.B. Bolin, and A.I. Zegna (1988) Optimization of synthesis of pyridoxylated polymerized stroma-free hemoglobin solution. *Milit Med* 153:1–44.

Mason, A.D., and C.B. Mueller (1952) Experimental observations on the role played by anaphylaxis in the development of renal disease following the infusion of mismatched blood. *Science* 116:526.

Mason, J.B., and F.C. Mann (1931) The effect of hemoglobin on volume of the kidney. *Am J Physiol* 98:181–85.

Matsushita, M., A. Yabuki, P.S. Malchesky, H. Harasaki, and Y. Nose (1988) In vivo evaluation of a pyridoxylated-hemoglobin-polyoxyethylene conjugate. *Biomater Artif Cells Artif Organs* 16:247–60.

Mazur, A., S. Baez, and E. Shorr (1955) The mechanism of iron release from ferritin as related to its biological properties. *J Biol Chem* 213:147–60.

Mazur, A., S. Green, A. Saha, and A. Carleton (1958) Mechanism of release of ferritin iron in vivo by xanthine oxidase. *J Clin Invest* 37:1809–17.

McCord, J.M. (1985) Oxygen-derived free radicals in postischemic tissue injury. *N Engl J Med* 312:159–63.

McCormack, L.R., H.H. Liem, W.B. Strum, S.M. Grundy, and U. Muller-Eberhard (1982) Effects of haem infusion on biliary secretion of porphyrins, haem, and bilirubin in man. *Eur J Clin Invest* 12:257–62.

McDonald, R.K., J.H. Miller, and E.B. Roach (1951) Human glomerular permeability and tubular recovery values for hemoglobin. *J Clin Invest* 30:1041–45.

McGarrity, M.J., S.S. Er, and J.C. Hsia (1987) Hemoglobin-based blood substitutes: Characterization of five pyridoxal 5'-phosphate derivatives of hemoglobin. *J Chromatogr* 419:1–14.

McGarrity, M.J., S.S. Er, K.A. Nightingale, and J.C. Hsia (1987) Isolation and partial characterization of pyridoxal 5'-phosphate hemoglobins by high performance liquid chromatography as a quality control method for hemoglobin-based blood substitutes. *J Chromatogr* 413:53–63.

McGarrity, M.J., K.A. Nightingale, and J.C. Hsia (1987) ATP-hemoglobin: Anomalous oxygen binding properties. *J Chromatogr, Biomed Appl* 415:136–42.

McPherson, J.M., S. Sawamura, and R. Armstrong (1986) An examination of the biologic response to injectable, glutaraldehyde cross-linked collagen implants. *J Biomed Mater Res* 20:93–107.

Menefee, M.G., C.B. Mueller, T.B. Miller, J.K. Meyers, and A.L. Bell (1964) Experimental studies in acute renal failure. II. Fine structure changes in tubules associated with renal failure induced by globin. *J Exp Med* 120:1139–49.

Menitove, J. (1989) The decreasing risk of transfusion-associated AIDS. *N Engl J Med* 321:966–68.

Menu, P., F. Pauly, P. Labrude, and C. Vigneron (1987) Haemoglobin pyridoxylation: Optimization and observation of an additional new pyridoxal phosphate-haemoglobin species by high performance liquid chromatographic resolution. *J Chromatogr* 417:397–402.

Menu, P., P. Voisin, P. Labrude, and C. Vigneron (1985) Total exchange transfusion in rats with hemoglobin solutions: Influence of hemoglobin concentration. *Int J Artif Org* 8:341–45.

Messmer, K. (1988) Characteristics, effects and side-effects of plasma substitutes. In *Blood Substitutes. Preparation Physiology and Medical Applications* (K.C. Lowe, ed) 51–70, Chichester: Ellis Horwood.

Miller, D.M., R.M. Winslow, H.G. Klein, K.C. Wilson, F.L. Brown, and N.J. Statham (1980) Improved exercise performance after exchange transfusion in subjects with sickle-cell anemia. *Blood* 56:1127–31.

Miller, F. (1960) Hemoglobin absorption by the cells of the proximal convoluted tubule in mouse kidney. *J Biophys Biochem Cytol* 8:689–718.

Miller, J.H., and R.K. McDonald (1951) The effect of hemoglobin on renal function in the human. *J Clin Invest* 30:1033–40.

Miller, J.R., and C.A. Poindexter (1932) The effects observed following the intravenous and subcutaneous administration of fluid: An experimental study on dogs. *J Lab Clin Med* 18:287–97.

Misra, H.P., and I. Fridovich (1972) The generation of superoxide radical during the autoxidation of hemoglobin. *J Biol Chem* 247:6960–62.

Miyamoto, K., E. Schultz, T. Heath, M. Mitchell, K.H. Albertine, and N.C. Staub (1988) Pulmonary intravascular macrophages and hemodynamic effects in sheep. *J Appl Physiol* 64:1143–52.

Miyamoto, K., E. Schultz, M. Mitchell, and N.C. Staub (1987) Systemic arterial thromboxane concentrations after liposome infusions in three species with pulmonary intracapillary macrophages. *Fed Proc* 46:1109.

Miyamoto, K., E. Schultz, and N.C. Staub (1977) Pulmonary vascular response and lung uptake of liposomes in seven animal species. *Physiologist* 29:177 (abstr).

Modig, J. (1983) Advantages of dextran 70 over Ringer acetate solution in shock treatment and in prevention of adult respiratory distress syndrome: A randomized study in man after traumatic-haemorrhagic shock. *Resuscitation* 10:219–26.

Modig, J. (1986) Effectiveness of dextran 70 versus Ringer's acetate in traumatic shock and adult respiratory distress syndrome. *Crit Care Med* 14:454–57.

Mohanty, M., T.V. Kumari, K. Rathinam, and Vijayakumari (1989) Pulmonary vasospasm in rabbits infused with stroma free hemoglobin solution. *Indian J Exp Biol* 27:265–68.

Mok, W., D.E. Chen, and A. Mazur (1975) Cross-linked hemoglobins as potential plasma expanders. *Fed Proc* 34:1458–60.

Moldovan, J. (1910) Über die Wirkung intravaskularer Injektionen frischen, defibrinierten Blutes und ihre Beziehungen zur Frage der Transfusion. *Dtsch Med Wochenschr* 2:2422–25.

Mollison, P.L. (1983) *Blood Transfusion in Clinical Medicine,* 7th ed Philadelphia: FA Davis.

Monod, J., J. Wyman, and J. Changeaux (1965) On the nature of allosteric transitions: A plausible model. *J Mol Biol* 12:88–118.

Moore, G.L., M.E. Ledford, and J.A. Tillotson (1986) Molecular heterogeneity of pyridoxylated polymerized hemoglobin. San Francisco: Letterman Army Institute of Research Report 227.

Moores, W.Y., F. DeVenuto, W.H. Heydorn, A.G. Greenburg, and J.R. Utley (1982) Effectiveness of stroma-free hemoglobin solution as seen in a right heart bypass in swine. *Crit Care Med* 10:279–82.

Morgan, W.T., H.H. Liem, R.P. Sutor, and U. Muller-Eberhard (1976) Transfer of heme from heme-albumin to hemopexin. *Biochim Biophys Acta* 444:435–45.

Morimoto, H., H. Lehmann, and M.F. Perutz (1971) Molecular pathology of human hemoglobin: Stereochemical interpretation of abnormal oxygen affinity. *Nature* 232:408–13.

Morris, D.L., M.D. Dudley, and R.D. Pearson (1981) Coagulopathy associated with hematin treatment for acute intermittent porphyria. *Ann Intern Med* 95:700–1.

Morrison, A.R. (1986) Biochemistry and pharmacology of renal arachidonic acid metabolism. *Am J Med* 80:3–11.

Morrison, A.R., J.E. Benabe, and M.K. Hoffman (1980) Identification of thromboxane A_2 in glycerol-induced acute renal failure in the rabbit. *Adv Prostaglandin Thromboxane Res* 7:1131–33.

Mosebar, R.H. (1989) Military uses of oxygen carrying resuscitation fluids. *Biomater Artif Cells Artif Organs* 17:6.

Moss, G.S., R. De Woskin, A.L. Rosen, H. Levine, and C.K. Palani (1976) Transport of oxygen and carbon dioxide by hemoglobin-saline solution in the red cell free primate. *Surg Gynecol Obstet* 142:357–62.

Moss, G.S., S.A. Gould, A.L. Rosen, L.R. Sehgal, and H.L. Sehgal (1989) Results of the first clinical trial with a polymerized hemoglobin solution. *Biomater Artif Cells Artif Organs* 17:633.

Moss, G.S., S.A. Gould, L.R. Sehgal, H.L. Sehgal, and A.L. Rosen (1988) Hemoglobin solution: From tetramer to polymer. *Biomater Artif Cells Artif Organs* 16:57–69.

Mudd, S. (1942) Recapitulation and outlook. In *Blood Substitutes and*

Blood Transfusion (S. Mudd and W. Thalhimer, eds) 291–299, Springfield, Ill.: Charles C Thomas.

Mulder, A.G., W.R. Amberson, F.R. Steggerda, and J. Flexner (1934) Oxygen consumption with hemoglobin-Ringer. *J Cell Comp Physiol* 5:383–97.

Muller-Eberhard, U. (1970) Hemopexin. *N Engl J Med* 283:1090–94.

Muller-Eberhard, U., and H. Nikkila (1989) Transport of tetrapyrroles by proteins. *Semin Hematol* 26:86–104.

Munakata, M., W. Mitzner, and H. Menkes (1988) Osmotic stimuli induce epithelial-dependent relaxation in the guinea pig trachea. *J Appl Physiol* 64:466–71.

National Institutes of Health Consensus Conference (1988) Perioperative red cell transfusion. *JAMA* 260:2700–3.

Neely, S.M., D.V. Gardner, N. Reynolds, D. Green, and C.H. Ts'o (1984) Mechanism and characteristics of platelet activation by hematin. *Br J Haematol* 58:305–16.

Nemeth, I., and D. Boda (1989) The ratio of oxidized/reduced glutathione as an index of oxidative stress in various experimental models of shock syndrome. *Biochim Biophys Acta* 48:53–57.

Neville, J.R. (1976) Altered haem-haem interaction and tissue–oxygen supply: A theoretical analysis. *Br J Haematol* 34:387–95.

Nicolson, M.H. (1965) *Pepys' Diary and the New Science*. Charlottesville: University Press of Virginia.

Ning, J., and Chang, T.M.S. (1990) In vivo effects of stroma-free hemoglobin and polyhemoglobin on coagulation factors in rats. *Int J Artif Organs* 13:509–16.

Nitta, S., T. Ohnuki, T. Nakada, and N.C. Staub (1981) The corrected protein equation to estimate plasma colloid osmotic pressure and its development on a nomogram. *Tohoku J Exp Med* 135:43–49.

O'Mara, P.A., R.A. Patterson, G.E. Esgandarin, F. DeVenuto, and P.W. Mellick (1978) Behavioral effects of massive transfusions with cell-free resuscitating solutions. San Francisco: Letterman Army Institute of Research Report 45.

Oberman, H.A. (1969) Early history of blood transfusion: Transfusion of milk. *Transfusion* 9:74–7.

Odling-Smee, W., and C. McLarnon (1984) Haemoglobin solution as an oxygen-carrying resuscitation fluid in haemorrhagic shock. *Irish J Med Sci* 153:385–88.

Oken, D.E., M.L. Arce, D.R. Wilson (1966) Glycerol-induced hemoglobinuric acute renal failure in the rat. I. Micropuncture study of the development of oliguria. *J Clin Invest* 45:724–35.

Oliver, J., M. MacDowell, and Y.C. Lee (1954) Cellular mechanisms of protein metabolism in the nephron. I. The structural aspects of proteinuria, tubular absorption, droplet formation, and the disposal of proteins. *J Exp Med* 99:589–604.

Olson, J.S., A.J. Mathews, B.A. Springer, K.D. Egeberg, S.G. Sligar, J. Tame, J.P. Renaud, and K. Nagai (1988) The role of the distal histidine in myoglobin and haemoglobin. *Nature* 336:265–66.

O'Shaughnessy, L., H.E. Mansell, and D. Slome (1939) Haemoglobin solution as a blood substitute. *Lancet* 2:1068–69.

Ottenberg, R., and C.L. Fox (1938) The rate of removal of hemoglobin from the circulation and its renal threshold in human beings. *Am J Physiol* 123:516–25.

Palani, C.K., R. DeWoskin, M. Michuda, A.L. Rosen, and G.S. Moss (1974) In vivo oxygen transport with a stroma-free hemoglobin solution in primates. *Surg Forum* 25:199–201.

Paller, M.S. (1988) Hemoglobin- and myoglobin- induced acute renal failure in rats: Role of iron in nephrotoxicity. *Am J Physiol* 253:F539–44.

Paller, M.S., B.E. Hedlund, J.J. Sikora, A. Faasen, and R. Waterfield (1988) Role of iron in postischemic renal injury in the rat. *Kidney Int* 34:474–80.

Payne, J.W. (1973) Polymerization of proteins with glutaraldehyde. Soluble molecular-weight markers. *Biochem J* 135:867–73.

Penfield, W.G. (1919) The treatment of severe and profusive hemorrhage by intravenous injection. *Amer J Physiol* 49:121–320.

Pennell, R.B., and W.E. Smith (1949) Preparation of stabilized solutions of hemoglobin. *Blood* 4:380–94.

Perrella, M. (1988) Intermediate compounds between hemoglobin and CO under equilibrium and kinetic conditions. *Symposium on Oxygen Binding Heme Proteins*, 8, Pacific Grove, Calif. (Asilomar).

Perrella, M., and L. Rossi-Bernardi (1981) Measurement of CO_2 equilibria: The chemical-chromatographic methods. *Methods Enzymol 76:*487–495.

Perutz, M.F. (1989) Myoglobin and haemoglobin: Role of distal residues in reactions with haem ligands. *Trends Biochem Sci* 14:42–44.

Peskin, G.W., K. O'Brien, and S.F. Rabiner (1969) Stroma-free haemoglobin solution: the "ideal" blood substitute? *Surgery* 66:185–93.

Phillips, R.A., V.P. Dole, P.B. Hamilton, K. Emerson, R.M. Archibald, and D.D. VanSlyke (1946) Effects of acute hemorrhagic and traumatic shock on renal function of dogs. *Am J Physiol* 145:314–36.

Phillips, R.A., R. Gilder, J.H. Killough, G.B. Magill, and R.C. Smith (1951) The results of sixty-two large-volume hemoglobin infusions in man. Unpublished data.

Pristoupil, T.I., M. Kramlova, and T. Marik (1989) Hydrodynamic instability of "stroma-free" hemoglobin. *Biomater Artif Cells Artif Organs* 17:335–39.

Prough, D.S., J.C. Johnson, D.A. Stump, E.H. Stullken, G.V. Poole, and

G. Howard (1986) Effects of hypertonic saline versus lactated Ringer's solution on cerebral oxygen transport during resuscitation from hemorrhagic shock. *J Neurosurg* 64:627–32.

Przybelski, R.J., G.J. Kant, M.J. Bounds, M.V. Slayter, and R.M. Winslow (1990) Rat maze performance after resuscitation with cross-linked hemoglobin solution. *J Lab Clin Med* 115:579–88.

Przybelski, R.J., G.J. Kant, J.R. Leu, M.J. Bounds, and R.M. Winslow (1989) The effect of infusion of cross-linked hemoglobin solution on rat maze performance. *Biomater Artif Cells Artif Organs* 17:583–96.

Rabiner, S.F. (1975) Hemoglobin solution as a plasma expander. *Fed Proc* 34:1454–57.

Rabiner, S.F., J.R. Helbert, H. Lopas, and L.H. Friedman (1967) Evaluation of stroma-free haemoglobin for use as a plasma expander. *J Exp Med* 126:1127–42.

Rabiner, S.F., K. O'Brien, G.W. Peskin, and L.H. Friedman (1970) Further studies with stroma-free hemoglobin solution. *Ann Surg* 171:615–22.

Rabinovici, R., A.S. Rudolph, and G. Feuerstein (1989) Characterization of hemodynamic, hematologic, and biochemical responses to administration of liposome-encapsulated hemoglobin in the conscious, freely moving rat. *Circ Shock* 29:115–32.

Reid, W.L. (1929) Changes in the volume of the kidney in the intact animal. A plethysmographic study with especial reference to diuretics. *Am J Physiol* 90:157–67.

Relihan, M., and M.S. Litwin (1972) Effects of stroma-free haemoglobin solutions on clearance rate and renal function. *Surgery* 71:395–99.

Relihan, M., and M.S. Litwin (1973) Clearance rate and renal effects of stroma-free hemoglobin on acidotic dogs. *Surg Gynecol Obstet* 137:73–79.

Remuzzi, G., L. Imberti, M. Rossini, C. Morelli, C. Carminati, G.M. Cattaneo, and T. Bertani (1985) Increased glomerular thromboxane synthesis as a possible cause of proteinuria in experimental nephrosis. *J Clin Invest* 75:94–101.

Ringer, S. (1885) Regarding the influence of the organic constituents of the blood on the contractility of the ventricle. *J Physiol* 6:361–81.

Robert, C.H., L. Fall, and S.J. Gill (1988) Linkage of organic phosphates to oxygen binding in human hemoglobin at high concentrations. *Biochemistry* 27:6835–43.

Roger, H. (1919) Action comparative du sang hémolysé et du sang autolysé. *Comp Rend Soc Biol* 82:609.

Romanosky, A.J., M.E. Giaimo, R.E. Shepherd, and A.H. Burns (1986) The effect of in vivo endotoxin on myocardial function in vitro. *Circ Shock* 19:1–12.

Rose, M.Y., R.A. Thompson, W.R. Light, and J.S. Olson (1985) Heme transfer between phospholipid membranes and uptake by apohemoglobin. *J Biol Chem* 260:6632–40.

Rosen, A.L., L.R. Sehgal, S.A. Gould, H.L. Sehgal, and G.S. Moss (1986) Methodology to assess the oxygen concentration of red cells and stroma-free hemoglobin solutions. *Crit Care Med* 14:147–50.

Rosoff, C.B., and C.W. Walter (1952) The controlled laboratory production of hemoglobinuric nephrosis. *Ann Surg* 135:324–31.

Rossen, J.D., S.R. Snyder, R.E. Kerber, M.L. Marcus, and J.A. Walder (1987) Coronary perfusion with a modified hemoglobin prevents myocardial dysfunction during coronary occlusion. *Midwest AFCR Cardiovasc* 4:837 (abstr).

Roughton, F.J.W., E.C. DeLand, J.C. Kernohan, and J.W. Severinghaus (1972) Some recent studies of the oxyhemoglobin dissociation curve of human blood under physiological conditions and the fitting of the Adair equation to the standard curve. In *Oxygen Affinity of Hemoglobin and Red Cell Acid Base Status* (P. Astrup and M. Rørth, eds) 73–83, Copenhagen: Munksgaard.

Rozich, J.D., and R.V. Paul (1989) Acute renal failure precipitated by elevated colloid osmotic pressure. *Am J Med* 87:358–60.

Rush, B.F., J.A. Redan, J.J. Flanagan, J.B. Heneghan, J. Hsieh, T.F. Murphy, S. Smith, and G.W. Machiedo (1989) Does bacteremia observed in hemorrhagic shock have clinical significance? *Ann Surg* 210:342–47.

Sadrzadeh, S.M.H., E. Graf, S. Panter, P.E. Hallaway, and J.W. Eaton (1984) Hemoglobin: A biological Fenton reagent. *J Biol Chem* 259:14354–56.

Salari, J., and M.J.A. Walker (1989) Cardiac dysfunction caused by factors released from endotoxin-activated macrophages. *Circ Shock* 27:263–72.

Salaskin, S., and J. Kriwsky (1931) Untersuchungen uber die Harnstoffbildung im Tierkorper. III. Mitteilung. B. Perfusionsversuche. *Z Physiol Chem* 196:121–39.

Saltman, P. (1989) Oxidative stress: A radical review. *Semin Hematol* 26:249–56.

San George, R.C., and H.D. Hoberman (1986) Reaction of acetaldehyde with hemoglobin. *J Biol Chem* 261:6811–21.

Savitsky, J.P., J. Doczi, J. Black, and J.D. Arnold (1978) A clinical safety trial of stroma-free hemoglobin. *Clin Pharmacol Ther* 23:73–80.

Scannon, P.J. (1982) Molecular modifications of hemoglobin. *Crit Care Med* 10:261–65.

Schmidt, K. (1979) Polyvinylpyrrolidon-gebundenes Hämoglobin als ein Sauerstoff übertragender Blutersatstoff. *Klin Wochenschr* 57:1169–75.

Schmidt, P.J., and P.V. Holland (1967) Pathogenesis of the acute renal failure associated with incompatible transfusion. *Lancet* 2:1169–72.

Schuschereba, S.T., H.I. Friedman, F. DeVenuto, and E.S. Beatrice (1983) Morphological effects on the retina of massive exchange transfusion with stroma-free hemoglobin solution. *Lab Invest* 48:339–52.

Sehgal, L., A.L. Rosen, S. Gould, H. Sehgal, L. Dalton, J. Mayoral, and G. Moss (1979) In vitro and in vivo characteristics of polymerized pyridoxylated hemoglobin solution. *Fed Proc* 39:718 (abstr).

Sehgal, L.R., S.A. Gould, A.L. Rosen, H.L. Sehgal, and G.S. Moss (1984) Polymerized pyridoxylated hemoglobin: A red cell substitute with normal oxygen capacity. *Surgery* 95:433–38.

Sehgal, L.R., A.L. Rosen, S.A. Gould, H.L. Sehgal, and G.S. Moss (1986) Characteristics and efficacy of polymerized hemoglobin. Thirty-ninth ACEMB, 78, Baltimore, Md.

Sehgal, L.R., A.L. Rosen, G. Noud, H.L. Sehgal, S.A. Gould, R. DeWoskin, C.L. Rice, and G.S. Moss (1981) Large-volume preparation of pyridoxylated hemoglobin with high P_{50}. *J Surg Res* 30:14–20.

Sellards, A.W., and G.R. Minot (1916) Injection of hemoglobin in man and its relation to blood destruction, with especial reference to the anemias. *J Med Res* 34:469–94.

Shah, D.M., M.E. Gottleib, R.L. Rahm, H.H. Stratton, P.S. Barie, W.H. Paloski, and J.C. Newell (1982) Failure of red blood cell transfusion to increase oxygen transport or mixed venous PO_2 in injured patients. *J Trauma* 22:741–46.

Shepherd, R.E., K.H. McDonough, and A.H. Burns (1986) Mechanism of cardiac dysfunction in hearts from endotoxin-treated rats. *Circ Shock* 19:371–84.

Shulman, N.R., R.S. Weinrach, E.P. Libre, and H.L. Andrews (1965) The role of the reticuloendothelial system in the pathogenesis of idiopathic thrombocytopenic purpura. *Trans Assoc Am Physicians* 78:374–90.

Simoni, J., M. Feola, R. Tran, M. Buckner, P.C. Canizaro (1990) Biocompatibility of hemoglobin solutions. II. The inflammatory reaction of human monocytes and mouse peritoneal macrophages. *Artif Organs* 14:98–109.

Sloviter, H.A., and T. Kamimoto (1967) Erythrocyte substititutes for perfusion of brain. *Nature* 216:458–60.

Sloviter, H.A., B. Mukherji, R. Benesch, R.E. Benesch, and S. Kwong (1981) Persistence of intradimerically cross-linked hemoglobin in rat plasma. *Fed Proc* 42:652.

Smith, C.D., S.T. Schuschereba, J.R. Hess, L. McKinney, D. Bunch, and P.D. Bowman (1990) Liver and kidney injury after administration of hemoglobin cross-linked with bis(3,5-dibromosalicyl)fumarate. *Biomater Artif Cells Artif Organs* 18:251–62.

Smith, D.J., and R.M. Winslow (1991) Effects of extraerythrocytic hemoglobin and its components on mononuclear cell procoagulant activity.

J Lab Clin Med in press.

Smith, G.J., G.C. Kramer, P. Perron, S.I. Nakayama, R.A. Gunther, and J.W. Holcroft (1985) A comparison of several hypertonic solutions for resuscitation of bled sheep. *J Surg Res* 39:517–28.

Smith, H.W. (1951) *The Kidney: Structure and Function in Health and Disease.* New York: Oxford University Press.

Snyder, S.R., E.V. Welty, R.Y. Walder, L.A. Williams, J.A. Walder (1987) A hemoglobin derivative that is cross-linked between the α subunits is useful as a blood substitute. *Proc Natl Acad Sci USA* 84:7280–84.

Spector, J.I., and W.H. Crosby (1975) Coagulation studies during experimental hemoglobinemia in humans. *J Appl Physiol* 38:195–98.

Speer, D.P., M. Chvapil, C.D. Eslekson, and J. Ulreich (1980) Biologic effects of residual glutaraldehyde in glutaraldehyde-tanned collagen biomaterials. *J Biomed Mater Res* 14:753–64.

Stainsby, W.N., and A.B. Otis (1964) Blood flow, oxygen tension and oxygen transport in skeletal muscle. *Am J Physiol* 206:858–66.

Starling, E.H. (1896) On the absorption of fluids from the connective tissue spaces. *J Physiol Lond* 19:312–26.

Starnes, H.F., A. Tewari, K. Flokas, J.C. Kosek, D. Brown, A.L. VanKessel, and C.E. Mondon (1991) Effectiveness of a purified human hemoglobin as a blood substitute in the perfused rat liver. *Gastroenterology*, submitted for publication.

Staub, N.C. (1988) Pulmonary intravascular macrophages. *Chest* 93:84s–85s.

Steinau, U., and O. Elert (1980) Prolongation of the ischemia tolerance of amputated extremities by a stroma-free hemoglobin solution. *Thorac Cardiovasc Surg* 28:35.

Suffredini, A.F., R.E. Fromm, M.M. Parker, M. Brenner, J.A. Kovacs, R.A. Wesley, and J.E. Parrillo (1989) The cardiovascular response of normal humans to the administration of endotoxin. *N Engl J Med* 321:280–87.

Surgenor, D.M., E.L. Wallace, S.G. Hale, and M.W. Gilpatrick (1988) Changing patterns of blood transfusions in four sets of United States hospitals, 1980 to 1985. *Transfusion* 28:513–18.

Tam, S.C., J. Blumenstein, and J.T.F. Wong (1976) Soluble dextran-hemoglobin complex as a potential blood substitute. *Proc Natl Acad Sci USA* 73:2128–2131.

Tam, S.C, J. Blumenstein, and J.T.F. Wong (1978) Blood replacement in dogs by dextran-hemoglobin. *Can J Biochem* 56:981–84.

Tam, S.C., and J.T.F. Wong (1988) Impairment of renal function by stroma-free hemoglobin in rats. *J Lab Clin Med* 111:189–93.

Tewari, A., C.E. Mondon, D. Brown, A.L. VanKessel, J.C. Kosek, and H.F. Starnes (1990) Proposed use of cross-linked hemoglobin as a blood substitute. *Surg Forum* 41:315–17.

Thomas, T.G. (1878) The intravenous injection of milk as a substitute for the transfusion of blood. *NY State J Med* 27:449–65.

Triner, L., R. Benesch, R.E. Benesch, S. Kwong, and M. Verosky (1983) The rate of plasma clearance of cross-linked and pyridoxylated hemoglobin in the rat. *Physiologist* 26:69(abstr).

Tsuchida, E., D. Eng, and H. Nishide (1988) Liposome/heme as a totally synthetic oxygen carrier. *Biomater Artif Cells Artif Organs* 16:313–19.

Tye, R.W., F. Medina, R.B. Bolin, G.L. Knopp, G.S. Irion, and S.K. McLaughlin (1983) Modification of hemoglobin: Tetrameric stabilization. In *Progress in Clinical and Biological Research: Advances in Blood Substitute Research* (R.B. Bolin, R.P. Geyer, and G.J. Nemo, eds) 41–49, New York: Alan R. Liss.

Vandegriff, K., and J.S. Olson (1984) Morphological and physiological factors affecting the oxygen uptake and release by red blood cells. *J Biol Chem* 259:12619–27.

Vandegriff, K.D., L. Benazzi, M. Ripamonti, M. Perrella, Y.C. LeTellier, A. Zegna, and R.M. Winslow (1991) Carbon dioxide binding to hemoglobin cross-linked between the α chains. *J Biol Chem* 266:2697–2700.

Vandegriff, K.D., F. Medina, M.A. Marini, and R.M. Winslow (1989) Equilibrium oxygen binding to human hemoglobin cross-linked between the α chains by bis(3,5-dibromosalicyl)fumarate. *J Biol Chem* 264:17824–33.

VanderPlas, J., J.B.L. Damm, and J.C. Bakker (1987) Preparation and physical characteristics of a hemoglobin solution modified by coupling to 2-nor-2-formylpyridoxal 5'- phosphate. *Transfusion* 27:425–30.

VanderPlas, J., A. DeVries-Van Rossen, W.K. Bleeker, and J.C. Bakker (1986) Effect of coupling of 2-nor-2-formylpyridoxal 5'- phosphate to stroma-free hemoglobin on oxygen affinity and tissue oxygenation: Studies in the isolated perfused rat liver under conditions of normoxia and stagnant hypoxia. *J Lab Clin Med* 108:253–60.

van Holde, K.E., and E.F.J. van Bruggen (1971) The hemocyanins. *Subunits Biol Syst* 5:1–53.

Vedder, N.B., B.W. Fouty, R.K. Winn, J.M. Harlan, and C.L. Rice (1989) Role of neutrophils in generalized reperfusion injury associated with resuscitation from shock. *Surgery* 106:509–16.

Vincent, S.H. (1989) Oxidative effects of heme and porphyrins on proteins and lipids. *Semin Hematol* 26:105–13.

Vincent, S.H., R.W. Grady, N. Shaklai, J.M. Snider, and U. Muller-Eberhard (1988) The influence of heme-binding proteins in heme-catalyzed oxidations. *Arch Biochem Biophys* 265:539–50.

Vogel, W.M., R.C. Dennis, G. Cassidy, C.S. Apstein, and C.R. Valeri (1986) Coronary constrictor effect of stroma-free hemoglobin solutions. *Am J Physiol* 251:H413–20.

Vogel, W.M., W. Lieberthal, C.S. Apstein, N. Levinsky, and C.R. Valeri (1988) Effects of stroma-free hemoglobin solutions on isolated perfused rabbit hearts and isolated perfused rat kidneys. *Biomater Artif Cells Artif Organs* 16:227–35.

VonStark, G. (1898) Die Resorborbarkeit des Haimatins und die Bedeutungder Haemoglobin-preparate. *Dtsch Med Wochenschr* 24: 805–08.

Walder, J.A., R.Y. Walder, and A. Arnone (1980) Development of antisickling compounds that chemically modify hemoglobin S specifically within the 2,3-diphosphoglycerate binding site. *J Mol Biol* 141:195–216.

Walder, J.A., R.H. Zaugg, R.Y. Walder, J.M. Steele, and I.M. Klotz (1979) Diaspirins that cross-link α chains of hemoglobin: bis(3,5-dibromosalicyl) succinate and bis(3,5-dibromosalicyl)fumarate. *Biochemistry* 18:4265–70.

Wangensteen, O.H., H. Hall, A. Kremen, and B. Stevens (1940) Intravenous administration of bovine and human plasma to man: Proof of utilization. *Proc Soc Exp Biol Med* 43:616–21.

Ward, J.W., S.D. Holmberg, J.R. Allen, D.L. Cohn, S.E. Critchley, S.H. Kleinman, B.A. Lenes, O. Ravenholt, J.R. Davis, M.G. Quinn, and H.W. Jaffe (1988) Transmission of human immunodeficiency virus (HIV) by blood transfusion screened as negative for HIV antibody. *N Engl J Med* 318:473–78.

Wasserman, K., J.E. Hansen, and D.Y. Sue (1991) Facilitation of oxygen consumption by lactic acidosis during exercise. *News Physiol Sci* 6:29–34.

Watzek, C., and K. Steinbereithner (1988) O_2 transporting blood substitutes in hemorrhagic shock. *Biomater Artif Cells Artif Organs* 16:661–63.

Weary, M.E. (1990) Understanding and setting endotoxin limits. *J Parenter Sci Technol* 44:16–18.

Weber, G. (1982) Asymmetric ligand binding by haemoglobin. *Nature* 300:603–7.

Weiss, S.J. (1980) The role of superoxide in the destruction of erythrocyte targets by human neutrophils. *J Biol Chem* 255:9912–17.

Wever, R., B. Oudega, and B.F. VanGelder (1973) Generation of superoxide radicals during the autoxidation of mammalian oxyhemoglobin. *Biochim Biophys Acta* 302:475–78.

White, C.T., A.J. Murray, J.R. Greene, D.J. Smith, F. Medina, G. Makovec, and R.B. Bolin (1986) Toxicity of human hemoglobin solutions infused into rabbits. *J Lab Clin Med* 108:121–31.

White, C.T., A.J. Murray, D.J. Smith, J.R. Greene, and R.B. Bolin (1986) Synergistic toxicity of endotoxin and hemoglobin. *J Lab Clin Med* 108:132–37.

White, F.L., and K.W. Olsen (1987) Effects of cross-linking on the thermal stability of hemoglobin. *Arch Biochem Biophys* 258:51–57.

Willford, D.C., E.P. Hill, and W.V. Moores (1982) Theoretical analysis of optimal P_{50}. *J Appl Physiol* 52:1043–48.

Williams, G.A., and S.P. Kent (1981) Specific identification of hemoglobin and myoglobin in renal tubular casts by the fluorescent antibody technic on fixed embedded tissues. *Am J Clin Pathol* 75:726–30.

Wilson, W.A., and E.J. Thomas (1979) Activation of the alternate pathway of human complement by haemoglobin. *Clin Exp Immunol* 36:140–44.

Winslow, R.M. (1985) A model for red cell O_2 uptake. *Int J Clin Monit Comput* 2:81–93.

Winslow, R.M. (1989) Blood substitutes: Current status. *Transfusion* 29:753–54.

Winslow, R.M., and W.F. Anderson (1982) The hemoglobinopathies. In *The Metabolic Basis of Inherited Disease*, 5th ed (J.B. Stanbury, J.B. Wyngaarden, D.S. Frederickson, J.L. Goldstein, and M.S. Brown, eds) 1666–1710, New York: McGraw-Hill.

Winslow, R.M., and C.C. Monge (1987) *Hypoxia, Polycythemia, and Chronic Mountain Sickness*. Baltimore: The Johns Hopkins University Press.

Winslow, R.M., C.C. Monge, E.G. Brown, H.G. Klein, F. Sarnquist, and N.J. Winslow (1985) The effects of hemodilution on O_2 transport in high altitude polycythemia. *J Appl Physiol* 59:1495–1502.

Winslow, R.M., M. Samaja, and J.B. West (1984) Red cell function at extreme altitude on Mount Everest. *J Appl Physiol* 56:109–16.

Winslow, R.M., M. Samaja, N.J. Winslow, L. Rossi-Bernardi, and R.I. Shrager (1983) Simulation of the continuous O_2 equilibrium curve over the physiologic range of pH, 2,3-diphosphoglycerate, and PCO_2. *J Appl Physiol* 54:524–29.

Winslow, R.M., M.L. Swenberg, R.L. Berger, R.I. Shrager, M. Luzzana, M. Samaja, and L. Rossi-Bernardi (1977) Oxygen equilibrium curve of normal human blood and its evaluation by Adair's equation. *J Biol Chem* 252:2331–37.

Winslow, R.M., N.J. Winslow, and M. Samaja (1990) Determination of the Adair parameters for the oxygen equilibrium curve of whole human blood by analysis of the temperature effect. Unpublished observations.

Wong, J.T.F. (1988) Rightshifted dextran-hemoglobin as blood substitute. *Biomater Artif Cells Artif Organs* 16:237–45.

Wood, L.E., D.N. Haney, J.R. Patel, S.E. Clare, G.-Y. Shi, L.C. King, and I.M. Klotz (1981) Structural specificities in acylation of hemoglobin and sickle hemoglobin by diaspirins. *J Biol Chem* 256:7046–52.

Woodson, R.D., B. Wranne, and J.C. Detter (1973) Effect of increased blood oxygen affinity on work performance of rats. *J Clin Invest* 52:2717–24.

Wright, C.J. (1975) Blood flow and oxygen consumption during severe progressive hemodilution. *Surg Forum* 25:198–99.

Wu, X.F., L.S. Porter, and J.T.F. Wong (1989) Properties of oxidized inositol tetrakisphosphate-rightshifted hemoglobin and dextran-hemoglobin. *Biomater Artif Cells Artif Organs* 17:645.

Wyman, J. (1964) Linked functions and reciprocal effects in hemoglobins: a second look. In *Advances in Protein Chemistry* (C.B. Anfinson, M.L. Anson, J.T. Edsall, and F.M. Richards, eds) 223–286, New York: Academic Press.

Yamakawa, T., Y. Miyauchi, K. Nishi (1990) Effects of pyridoxylated hemoglobin polyoxyethylene conjugate and stroma-free hemoglobin on cardiac function in isolated rat heart. *Artif Organs* 14:208–17.

Yang, T., and K.W. Olsen (1988) Effects of cross-linking on the thermal stability of hemoglobins. *Arch Biochem Biophys* 261:283–90.

Zaugg, R.H., L.C. King, and I.M. Klotz (1975) Acylation of hemoglobin by succinyldisalicylate, a potential cross-linking reagent. *Biochem Biophys Res Commun* 64:1192–98.

Zhang, L., J.M. Rifkind, and A. Levy (1990) A perturbed "R" state responsible for hemoglobin oxidation. *Biophys J* 57:239 (abstr).

Zipser, R.D. (1985) Effects of selective inhibition of thromboxane synthesis on renal function in humans. *Am J Physiol* 248:F753–56.

Zuck, T.F. (1988) Editorial. Silent sequences and the safety of blood transfusions. *Ann Intern Med* 108:895–96.

Index

Robert M. Winslow, M.D., is Chief of the Blood Research Division, Letterman Army Institute of Research, and Adjunct Professor in the Department of Medicine at the University of California, San Diego. He earned an M.D. from the Johns Hopkins University School of Medicine and received further training at the Massachusetts Institute of Technology and the National Institutes of Health. His research has been related to hemoglobin, whether in basic biochemical mechanisms (the structure and function of mutant and modified hemoglobin), the physiology of oxygen transport (high-altitude physiology), or clinical applications (sickle cells anemia, polycythemia). His high-altitude work, carried out in the Andes of Peru and Chile and in the Himalayas, culminated in the publication of *Hypoxia, Polycythemia, and Chronic Mountain Sickness* (Johns Hopkins University Press, 1987), with Carlos Monge C. as co-author. From 1985 to 1991 Dr. Winslow directed studies of the biochemistry and physiology of hemoglobin-based red cell substitutes. In addition to this research, he has served as a consultant to the Federal Aviation Administration, the Food and Drug Administration, and the Pan American Health Organization.